MARILYN WATERS WRASMAN

Chairman
Special Education Department
Dixie Hollins High School
Pinellas County, Florida

DISABLED

*Designed for use with adolescents
and young adults*

Danville, Illinois 61832

Lessons for the Language Disabled

Library of Congress Catalog Card No. 79-65480

ISBN 0-8134-2085-7

To

RICHARD GREGG
RICHARD SANDERS
MARILYN SHARBAUGH

and the

PARKLAND STAFF

Professional Educators and Friends

CONTENTS

Introduction, xi

| SECTION 1. I AM A PERSON | 1 |

Each Student Can Demonstrate an Understanding of the Concept, "Person," 3

Each Student Can Describe His Own Appearance, 7

Each Student Can Describe Himself As a Person, 13

Each Student Can Describe a Classmate, 17

Each Student Can Identify Emotions Represented in Prints of Paintings, 21

Each Student Can Verbally Identify Emotions, 27

Each Student Can Verbalize a Personal Experience in Which an Emotion Was Involved, 31

Each Student Can Role Play a Story, Demonstrating Appropriate Emotional Responses to Given Situations, 35

Each Student Can Demonstrate an Understanding of the Concept, "Responsibility," in Regard to Himself, 39

| SECTION 2. I AM A FAMILY MEMBER | 43 |

Each Student Can Demonstrate an Understanding of the Concept, "Family," 45

Each Student Can Identify Pictures of Family Members, 49

Each Student Can Identify Immediate Family Relationships, 53

Each Student Can Non-verbally Identify Extended Family Relationships Represented in Pictures, 59

Each Student Can Describe a Family Member, 65

Each Student Can Verbally Identify Extended Family Relationships, 69

Each Student Can Express Family Relationships in Sentences, 75

Each Student Can Complete a Story Involving a Family, 81

Each Student Can Tell a Story About Family Members Doing Something Together, 85

Each Student Can Demonstrate an Understanding of the Concept, "Responsibility," in Regard to His Own Family, 89

Each Student Can Demonstrate an Understanding of the Concept, "Responsibility," in Regard to Forming His Own Family Unit, 95

SECTION 3. I AM A WORKER   99

Each Student Can Demonstrate an Understanding of the Concept, "Work," 101

Each Student Can Identify Occupations Depicted in Pictures, 107

Each Student Can Demonstrate an Understanding of Work-related Vocabulary, 111

Each Student Can Identify Tasks Related to Different Occupations, 117

Each Student Can Describe a Work Experience, 123

Each Student Can Verbalize Skills Necessary for a Specific Job Available to Him, 129

Each Student Can Demonstrate an Understanding of the Procedures Necessary for Finding a Job, 133

Each Student Can Role Play a Job Interview, 139

Each Student Can Participate in a Problem-solving Situation Related to Work, 145

Each Student Can Demonstrate an Understanding of the Concept, "Responsibility," in Regard to Work, 151

| SECTION 4.   I AM A CONSUMER | 155 |

Each Student Can Demonstrate an Understanding of the
Concept, "Consumer," 157

Each Student Can Demonstrate an Understanding of
Consumer-related Vocabulary, 163

Each Student Can Verbalize Wise Shopping Habits, 169

Each Student Can Demonstrate an Understanding of a
Budget, 175

Each Student Can Demonstrate an Understanding of Consumer
Responsibilities, 181

Each Student Can Describe a Particular Product, 187

Each Student Can Role Play a Situation in Which a
Consumer-related Problem Is Solved, 193

| SECTION 5.   I AM A TRAVELER | 197 |

Each Student Can Demonstrate an Understanding of the
Concept, "Travel," 199

Each Student Can Demonstrate an Understanding of
Travel-related Vocabulary, 207

Each Student Can Verbalize a Travel Experience, 213

Each Student Can Demonstrate an Understanding of Procedures
Necessary for Planning a Trip, 217

Each Student Can Classify Items Appropriate to Particular
Vacation Areas, in Preparation for Traveling, 221

Each Student Can Verbalize Solutions to Problems That Might
Be Experienced While He Is Traveling, 227

Each Student Can Demonstrate an Understanding of the Concept,
"Safety," in Regard to Travel, 231

Each Student Can Verbalize in Simple Sentences Ways He Might
Show Courtesy to Others While He Is Traveling, 237

Each Student Can Demonstrate an Understanding of the Concept,
"Responsibility," in Regard to Travel, 243

INTRODUCTION

<u>LESSONS</u> <u>FOR</u> <u>THE</u> <u>LANGUAGE</u> <u>DISABLED</u> (<u>Designed</u> <u>for</u> <u>use</u> <u>with</u> <u>adolescents</u> <u>and</u> <u>young</u> <u>adults</u>) offers the teacher, therapist or parent a structured, sequential and systematic approach to developing and improving student listening, thinking and speaking skills.

As experienced language and speech therapists, the authors realized the need for guidelines for language disabled persons who required development of functional skills beyond the basic concepts.

<u>LESSONS</u> <u>FOR</u> <u>THE</u> <u>LANGUAGE</u> <u>DISABLED</u> is specifically designed for the adolescent and young adult, but it is not limited to this age group. Primary emphasis of the program should concentrate on language ability and need, rather than on the age level of the student. The program was used initially with mentally retarded adolescents and young adults in special education centers. These young people needed the development of practical language to assist them in functioning more effectively in their immediate environment. In assessing needs of students, the authors focused attention on student life styles as well as on general abilities. They developed a format which followed the student from his growth as an individual to his interaction as a functioning member of society.

The program has also proved to be effective when it has been used to develop language skills of students enrolled in basic language classes at the high school level.

This program adapts to the hearing impaired, the culturally disadvantaged and the student to whom English is a second language. It may be used by the teacher, therapist, parent or counselor as an important supplement to existing programs or as a primary reference source for home programs. Vocational and rehabilitation counselors can use it in conjunction with established training programs. The key to effective use of this program lies with the ability of the teacher to be aware of students' needs, strengths and weaknesses and to be able to adapt and modify the contents in order to best serve the students.

LESSONS FOR THE LANGUAGE DISABLED details 92 lesson plans geared to accomplishing 46 objectives. Materials necessary for each lesson are listed in a separate section preceding each activity. By using the checklist (page 2) to record students' progress, the teacher will be able to determine students' strengths and weaknesses. Of course, the teacher may modify the checklist in order to meet individual needs.

Procedures and instructions are written in simple language. Procedures are graded in level of difficulty, in order to enable the teacher to individualize lessons for classes composed of different ability ranges. For each objective, two procedures are presented. By modifying existing procedures, the teacher may use the lessons

to reinforce the material, in order to guide the student in accomplishing the objective.

The authors have provided teachers and parents with material for
developing functional language skills. These lessons provide
transitional material for the students who have mastered basic
concepts and are ready to develop advanced listening, thinking
and speaking skills.

HOW TO USE THE PROGRAM

The teacher may use the material in a number of ways. The final
decision on how to utilize the program best will ultimately lie
with the teacher. Students' needs will be the major determining
factor in establishing program guidelines and goals. Students'
needs will determine whether to present the material as a supplement to an existing language arts program, with the class participating as a whole; whether to use the material as a secondary
remediation program for small groups; or whether to use the material in conjunction with other professionals as a vehicle for rein-
forcing language skills.

If the program is presented to the class as a whole, the teacher
may wish to set aside approximately 50 minutes at least three
times a week for presentation.

If the program is used primarily with small groups of students,
the teacher may adjust the presentation time to 30-minute time
intervals twice weekly.

Although time limits and scheduling should remain flexible, definite time periods should be established for the activity.

The teacher may wish to collaborate with other professionals, using the material as a vehicle for reinforcement and carryover. Speech therapists, teachers of the hearing impaired or vocational counselors, for example, may wish to meet with the classroom teacher prior to initiation of the program. Specialists in the different areas may wish to discuss test results of students, pointing out specific skills which need to be developed. They may offer suggestions on how to supplement or modify the scope of the lesson plans in order to use them in conjunction with goals and objectives established in the remedial programs in which the students may be participating. If teaming is to be effective, the professionals involved should set aside specific times for meeting as a group to plan, to share ideas, to offer suggestions and to evaluate the effectiveness of the program.

In essence, the ability of the teacher to assess the needs of the students, to determine the most effective mode of delivery of the material and to generate a positive atmosphere for learning is the key ingredient in accomplishing the objectives detailed in LESSONS FOR THE LANGUAGE DISABLED.

ORGANIZATION

Once the teacher has determined how the material is to be used, has grouped the students and has established the time frame for lesson presentation, then he must determine the mechanics of organization.

MATERIALS

In reviewing the format of the lesson plans, one notes that each plan has a section entitled "Materials." It is suggested that the teacher set aside a particular area of the room for the storing of materials to be used in the presentation of the lessons. If the teacher plans to complete one objective in a week's time, the materials for two lesson plans should be stored in the area set aside for that purpose.

Once the materials have served their purpose, they may be stored in a large box or in a cabinet marked as to the number of the objective and the section in which the objective appears. This procedure should make it easier for the teacher to find materials should he be using the lesson plans with two or more groups which are working on different objectives.

Oftentimes, materials may be borrowed from parents or from colleagues. The authors have found it helpful to post a large piece of paper to the cabinet or to the box where materials are stored. On the paper, the teacher notes the name or the description of the material which has been borrowed, the person from whom the material was borrowed and the date the material was borrowed. This procedure should help to prevent loss of materials and embarrassment to the borrower.

Another area calling for organization is that of recording progress. A sample checklist is provided on page 2. Should the
teacher decide to use this format for recording student progress,
devising similar checklists for the remaining chapters will be
necessary. The checklist forms should be kept in a special folder
so that the information will be readily available to the teacher.
If the teacher decides to work in conjunction with other professionals, keeping notes from conferences or keeping test records
in a separate folder is helpful. Feedback from students concerning effectiveness of lessons, special problems and suggestions
should be kept on file. The teacher may wish to collect students'
notes, select certain comments to be retained and file these in a
separate envelope marked "Students' Comments." The teacher may
wish to keep a notebook on the desk for the purpose of jotting
down ideas, observations, informal evaluations and general data
which would be of interest to himself or to co-workers.

TEACHING TECHNIQUES

Reinforcement

The efforts of students to participate in task completion, as well
as the actual successful performance, should meet with reinforcement.

Primary reinforcement may consist of tangible rewards, such as
food, stars, achievement badges or so on.

Secondary reinforcement may consist of verbal or nonverbal ap-
proval from the teacher or from fellow students.

The teacher in initial lessons may use primary reinforcement for
all students and then gradually switch to secondary reinforcement
techniques. Some students may require more reinforcement than
others in order to establish and maintain motivational levels.

TEACHER-STUDENT INTERACTION

The following techniques are suggested for presenting the language
lessons:

1. The students should move at their own pace. The teacher may
deal with inappropriate or incomplete responses by rephrasing
directions in order to insure the student's understanding of
directions. If this is not effective, the teacher may wish to
provide the correct response, using simple language structure,
then have the student pattern the response. Further reinforcement
may be achieved by having another student answer the same question
and then by having the first student paraphrase the correct answer.
Of course, all attempts to complete tasks should be rewarded. If
progress continues to lag, the teacher may have to enlist the aid
of a speech pathologist, devise a tutoring program or provide the
parent with supportive materials to be used at home to reinforce
classroom work.

2. The teacher's attitude is as important as technique. Thus, the teacher should strive to be warm, friendly, responsive and objective.

EVALUATION

The teacher may wish to determine students' strengths, weaknesses and progress by systematically using the checklist format suggested by the authors or by developing another method of evaluation.

The goal of evaluation is to chart student progress systematically and objectively and to use the information gained to develop skills detailed in the program. Any method of evaluation that meets these requirements and is acceptable to the teacher should suffice.

SECTION 1

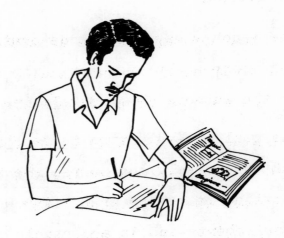

I Am a Person

SAMPLE CHECKLIST

Student

Each Student Can:	#1	#2	#3	#4	#5	#6	#7	#8
1. Demonstrate understanding of the concept, "person"								
2. Describe his own appearance								
3. Describe himself as a person								
4. Describe a classmate								
5. Identify emotions represented in pictures								
6. Verbally identify emotions ...								
7. Verbalize a personal experience in which an emotion was involved								
8. Role play a story, demonstrating appropriate emotional responses to given situations ...								

```
┌────────────────────────────────────────────────────────────────────┐
│  OBJECTIVE:  Each Student Can Demonstrate an Understanding of the Concept,  │
│              "Person"                                                │
└────────────────────────────────────────────────────────────────────┘
```

MATERIALS: Large pictures of persons, male and female, of
            different ages, races and nationalities; bulletin
            board; thumbtacks

PROCEDURE 1:

The students are seated in a semicircle, facing the bulletin
board. The teacher begins:

    Today we are going to talk about people. I
    have many pictures of people to show you. All
    the people in the pictures are different, but
    each one is a person. Everyone in this room
    looks different. Some of us are tall. Some
    of us are short. John is a tall person. I
    am a short person.

    John, stand next to me.

    See how different we are? We are different,
    but we are both persons.

    John, you may return to your place.

After John has been seated, the teacher continues:

    I am going to place some pictures of people
    on the board. You will see that the people
    in the pictures are different from us, but in
    many ways they are similar to us. They all

need food; they all need water; they all need
sleep; and they all have feelings. I will
put the pictures on the bulletin board. Find
the picture of a very old person.

After the pictures have been arranged on the bulletin board,
the teacher asks:

Pat, did you find the picture of a very old
person? If you did, come to the bulletin
board and point to the picture.

If Pat responds incorrectly, the teacher points to the picture of the old person and says:

This is a picture of a very old person. We
can tell that the person in the picture is
very old because her hair is white and her
skin is wrinkled.

You are young. Your hair is brown and your
skin is smooth. Now point to the picture of
the old person.

If Pat responds correctly, the teacher says:

Good, Pat. Let's look at the picture of the
old person. Even though this person is very
old, in many ways she is like you. How is
the person in the picture like you, Pat?
Yes, she is a female. Yes, she has a happy
smile. Yes, she wears glasses.

The teacher continues this activity, constantly emphasizing
that although the people depicted in the pictures have different characteristics, they are all people.

This activity continues until each student can demonstrate
an understanding of the concept, "person."

MATERIALS: Photos of people in Procedure 1; newsprint; felt-
             tipped pen; bulletin board; thumbtacks

PROCEDURE 2:

The students are seated in a semicircle, facing the bulletin
board. The teacher asks the students what the word "person"
means to them. Each student's response is recorded by the
teacher on a sheet of newsprint, which is attached to the
bulletin board. Ideas such as "a person can think";
"a person can know right from wrong"; "a person can plan
ahead" may be included in the students' responses.

The teacher continues:

> I am going to show you pictures of many peo-
> ple. These people may seem to be very dif-
> ferent from us. They dress differently.
> They eat different foods. They have differ-
> ent religions. They use different monies
> and live in different kinds of homes.

The teacher displays the photos on the bulletin board. Then
he initiates a discussion regarding the differences listed
above. In the discussion, the teacher uses, and explains,
new vocabulary words such as "tradition," "customs," and
"life-style."

The teacher remarks:

> We have talked about the ways in which the
> people in the pictures are different from us.
> In what ways are they similar to us?

The teacher asks for volunteers to explain how all people
are alike. As each student contributes information, the
teacher writes this information on the newsprint. (It is
very important for the teacher to convey the idea that all
people are alike in many ways but that they are also different in many ways; yet, all are persons.)

This activity continues until each student can demonstrate
an understanding of the concept, "person."

OBJECTIVE: Each Student Can Describe His Own Appearance

MATERIALS: Color photographs, one of each student; newsprint;
             felt-tipped pen; bulletin board; thumbtacks

PROCEDURE 1:

(Prior to this activity, the teacher should supply each
student with information concerning his height and weight.)

The students are seated in a semicircle, facing the bulletin
board. The teacher explains that each member of the group
will learn how to describe himself. He introduces the word
"description" and leads the group to the conclusion that "to
describe" is "to use words to form a picture" by explaining:

> This is a photo of Jeanne. I want each of you
> to look at it. Take the picture, look at it
> and then pass it to the classmate who is
> sitting next to you. After each of you has
> had a chance to look at it, I will put it on
> the bulletin board.

After each student has looked at the picture, the teacher
takes it and turns it so that the students cannot see it.
Then he says:

> Now that you cannot see the picture of Jeanne,
> I will tell how Jeanne looks in the picture.
> Jeanne has blue eyes. She has freckles. She
> is taller than I am. She has a pretty smile.

The teacher asks:

7

What did I forget in my description of
Jeanne?

Tom responds:

You forgot to say that Jeanne has red hair.

The teacher replies:

Yes, Tom, I forgot to say that Jeanne has red
hair. So, to help us remember what we need
for our word pictures or descriptions, I will
write some terms on our newsprint.

The teacher writes the following on the newsprint: "name,"
"age," "height," "color of eyes," "color of hair." Then the
teacher reads these to the class and comments:

I have a photograph of every member of the
class. I will look at each of your pictures
and use the words and phrases on the board to
help describe each of you.

Here is a picture of Ann. She is 15 years
old. She is tall. She weighs 105 pounds.
She has blue eyes. She has brown hair.

After the teacher has described each member of the class, by
using both the terms written on the newsprint and the
students' photographs, he asks:

Can you describe yourself? Can you use the
words on the newsprint to help form a picture
story about yourself? Tom, will you please
describe yourself for the class?

Tom responds:

My name is Tom Lee. I am 16 years old. I am
5'6". I weight 123 pounds. I have brown
eyes. I have brown hair.

8

The teacher replies:

> Good, Tom. You have described yourself for
> the class. You may keep your photograph.

This activity continues until each student can describe his
own appearance.

MATERIALS: Chalk; chalkboard; eraser

PROCEDURE 2:

(Prior to this activity, the teacher should take height and weight measurements for each student, explaining the words "height" and "weight," if necessary.)

The students are seated at their desks, facing the chalkboard. The teacher introduces the word "description" and lets the students define the term in their own words. Students' responses might include "to tell about something," "to form a word picture," etc.

The teacher lists the following terms: "name," "age," "height," "weight," "color of eyes," "color of hair," "sex" in a column on the chalkboard. Then, he explains:

> Look at the words which I have written on the board. Listen as I say the words for you. These words provide information about a person. Many times in our lives we must provide this information. When we apply for a job, when we open a bank account, when we apply for a driver's license, we must provide information about ourselves.
>
> Use the words on the board to give information about yourself. Cathy, use the words on the board to describe yourself.

Cathy responds:

Name:	Cathy Spicer is my name.
Age:	I am 15 years old.
Height:	I am 5'6".
Weight:	I weigh 109 pounds.
Color of eyes:	My eyes are brown.
Color of hair:	My hair is black.
Sex:	I am a female.

After Cathy has completed the description of herself, by using the words written on the board as a guideline, the teacher comments:

Good, Cathy. You have provided us with much information about yourself. You have described yourself.

The teacher then chooses another student to describe himself. This activity continues until each student can describe his own appearance.

OBJECTIVE: Each Student Can Describe Himself As a Person

MATERIALS: Photographs of students and one of the teacher; bulletin board; thumbtacks

PROCEDURE 1:

The students are seated in a semicircle, facing the bulletin board. On the bulletin board the teacher places photographs which were taken previously of the students at work.

The teacher explains:

> I have placed some photos of you on the bulletin board. I took these photos of you while you were working. I also have placed a picture of myself there. We can tell many things about ourselves from these pictures. Look at the one of me. What do you know about me from looking at it?
>
> Tom, tell the class what you know about me from looking at the picture.

Tom observes:

> You are a lady. You are tall. You wear glasses. You are thin.

The teacher continues:

Fine, Tom. You have told the class many
things about me. What do you know about me
that you do not see in the picture?

Tom responds:

You are nice. You like us.

The teacher replies:

Good, Tom. You may take the picture of yourself from the board. Tell us what you can
see in the picture.

Tom says:

I am tall. I am smiling. I am working.

The teacher continues:

Now tell us something about yourself that you
cannot see in the picture.

Tom responds:

I have four brothers. I am afraid of dogs.
I don't like people who laugh at me.

The teacher adds:

Now we know more about Tom. We know things
that we cannot see in the picture of Tom.
Each of you will have a chance to tell the
class two things about yourself that can be
seen in the picture of you on the board and
two things that cannot be seen in the picture.

This activity continues until each student can describe himself as a person.

MATERIALS: Five-part cutout of a person (on each part, one of
             the following is written: "Physical appearance,"
             "interests," "dislikes," "hobbies," "ambitions");
             bulletin board; thumbtacks

PROCEDURE 2:

   With the students seated at their desks, facing the bulletin
   board, the teacher begins:

        Today you are going to describe yourselves.
        Each of you will use terms to form a picture
        of yourself. On the bulletin board is a cut-
        out of a person. The cutout is divided into
        five parts. A term is written on each piece
        of the cutout. Listen as I read them.

   After the teacher has read the terms to the class, the
   teacher continues:

        When you tell about yourselves, you will use
        "special" words as a guide in describing
        yourselves as persons. The "special" words
        are written on the cutout of the person on
        the bulletin board. I will take the cutout
        apart now. I will tell you the term on each
        part of the cutout.

        The term on the first part of the cutout is
        "physical appearance." The physical appear-
        ance of a person is that part of the person
        that can be seen. Tonya, you may describe
        your physical appearance.

   If Tonya is unable to describe her physical appearance, the
   teacher says:

        We are going to help Tonya describe her
        physical appearance. Who can help us?

   After various students have responded, the teacher continues:

Tonya, John said that you are tall. Mary said
that your hair is red. Larry said that your
hair is curly. Tom told us that you have
freckles. Marie said that you have blue eyes.

Each of these students has helped to describe
your physical appearance. Now you may describe your physical appearance.

If Tonya is able to describe her physical appearance, the
teacher comments:

Good, Tonya. You have told the class how you
look. You have described your physical appearance. I will put that part of the cutout
which says "physical appearance" at the top
of the bulletin board.

The teacher then assists Tonya in describing herself as a
person, using the words written on the pieces of the cutout
as a guide. As Tonya describes herself as a person, according
to each category, the teacher adds a piece of the cutout until
the figure is completed.

The teacher praises Tonya, by remarking:

Well done, Tonya. You have described yourself
as a person. You have told about your physical appearance, interests, dislikes, hobbies
and ambitions. You have completed your cutout.
Would you like to tell us anything else about
yourself?

This activity continues until each student has had an opportunity to describe himself as a person.

OBJECTIVE: Each Student Can Describe a Classmate

MATERIALS: Photographs, one of each student, mounted separately
            on 8½" x 11" cardboard

PROCEDURE 1:

(Prior to this activity, the teacher has collected a photograph of each class member. Each photograph has been mounted
on an 8½" x 11" cardboard.)

The students are seated in a semicircle. The teacher
explains:

> Today you are going to describe your class-
> mates. I will give each of you a chance to
> tell about or to describe a person in the
> class. Each of you will be given a picture
> of a person in the class. Each of you will
> tell all you can about the person in the
> picture, but you cannot tell the person's
> name. When you have told all you can about
> the person in the picture, the other students
> will try to name that person.

The teacher selects a student to begin the activity and gives
the student one of the photographs. The teacher says:

> Leo, please go to the front of the class.
> Tell us as many things about this person in
> the picture as you can. Do not tell us the
> person's name.

17

After Leo has described the class member whose picture he is
holding, the teacher remarks:

> Good, Leo. You have told us many things about
> the person in your picture. You have de-
> scribed the person for us. Who can guess
> the name of the person?

After the person in the photograph has been identified, this
activity continues until each has had an opportunity to
describe a classmate.

MATERIALS: Chalk; chalkboard; eraser

PROCEDURE 2:

The students are seated at their desks, facing the chalkboard.
On the chalkboard, the teacher has written the following
words: "coloring," "sex," "age," "likes," "dislikes,"
"interests," "family." The teacher begins:

Today each of you will describe one of your
classmates. On the board, I have written
seven words. Listen as I point to them and
read them.

After the teacher has read the words to the class, the
teacher explains:

The seven words may be used as helpers in describing members of the class. I will now
use the words to describe one of our class
members. Listen carefully.

Coloring: This person has blue eyes and
                black hair.
                This person has light skin.

Sex: This person is a male.

Age: This person is 16 years old.

Likes: This person likes sports, es-
                pecially football.
                This person likes to sing.
                This person likes to dance.

Dislikes: This person does not like art.

Interests: This person is interested in
                working in a restaurant.
                This person is interested in
                learning how to become a salad
                maker in a restaurant.

Family: This person has two brothers, a
                mother and a father.

19

I have used the seven helping words to describe a member of the class. Who is this person?

After the class member has been identified, the teacher continues:

Marie, you may choose a class member to describe. Please do not tell the name of the class member. You may use the seven helping words on the board in describing the class member. When you have used all seven helping words, you may add anything else that you know about the person whom you are describing. Remember, do not tell the person's name.

This activity continues until each class member has had an opportunity to describe a classmate.

OBJECTIVE: Each Student Can Identify Emotions Represented in Prints of Paintings

MATERIALS: Art prints of people whose faces and posture demonstrate the emotions of joy, anger, surprise, fear (The school library may have prints of paintings, such as Norman Rockwell's Homecoming, Checkup, Game Called Because of Rain, available for the teacher's use.)

PROCEDURE 1:

The students are seated in a semicircle, facing the chalkboard. The teacher introduces the word "emotions" to the class and writes the word on the chalkboard. The teacher explains:

Emotion is the way someone or something makes us feel. If someone said to me, "You did a fine job on that bulletin board," I might feel proud and happy. These feelings of being proud and happy are emotions. I will write the words "pride," and "happiness" on our chalkboard under "emotions." While I write the words, think of who or what makes you feel proud and happy.

After writing the words on the board, the teacher continues:

If George said to me, "How could you make such a silly mistake?," how do you think I would feel, Ann?

Ann responds:

    You would feel sad.

The teacher replies:

    Yes, I might feel sad or angry or hurt. These
    feelings are all emotions. I will write these
    words on the board under "emotions," because
    they tell how I feel about someone or some-
    thing.

    Look at this picture. There are many people
    in this picture. We know what they are feeling
    by the expressions on their faces. John, what
    do you think the old man is feeling as he looks
    at the dog?

John responds:

    He looks angry.

The teacher agrees:

    Yes, John, he looks as though he is very
    angry. I think he is angry because he cannot
    move his truck. Ann, what do you think the
    little boy feels as he looks at the dog?

Ann answers:

    He looks scared.

The teacher concurs:

    Yes, Ann, he is afraid that the dog will be
    hurt. I am sure we all know what it is to
    feel angry and what it is to feel afraid.

The teacher uses the next three pictures, continuing the activity until each student has had an opportunity to identify emotions represented in the art prints.

MATERIALS: Same as in Procedure 1.

PROCEDURE 2:

The students are seated in a semicircle, facing the chalkboard. The teacher writes the word "emotions" on the chalkboard and explains:

> This word is "emotions." An "emotion" is the
> way we feel or react to a person or thing.
> Watch as I put my hand over the "E." Now the
> word is "motion." Many times a day our
> feelings are put into motion. We move from
> one feeling to another all day long.
>
> Suppose Ann woke up feeling very happy. Then,
> her mother said, "Ann, it's time to get up.
> Oh, Ann, this room is a mess! Look at your
> good skirt on the floor! You are old enough
> to take care of your things!"
>
> Ann's feelings go into action: they begin
> "to move." Ann might feel angry, hurt and
> guilty. These feelings she has are called
> "emotions." Let's name all the feelings we
> have experienced. I'll write them on the
> chalkboard as you think of them.

The teacher lists the emotions named by the students on the
board. The list may include love, anger, hate, joy, pride,
fear, loneliness, etc. He makes certain each student under-
stands the meaning of each of these words. He continues:

> Look at this picture. This picture is a
> favorite of mine because I can see how the
> people in the picture are feeling. Everyone
> in this picture reveals his feelings in his
> face or in his posture. However, we don't
> always show our feelings. Sometimes, it is
> hard to guess what someone is feeling.
>
> Les, as I point to each person in the picture,
> please tell us what you think that person is
> feeling.

After Les has identified the emotional reactions of each person depicted in the art print, the teacher asks the students to give the possible causes for the emotional reactions expressed by the persons in the print.

This activity continues until each student can identify emotions represented in the prints of paintings.

MATERIALS: Recordings featuring four current songs, each of which has as its theme one of the emotions: happiness, sadness, fear, surprise; four cartoon faces, each of which features one of the same emotions; bulletin board; thumbtacks

PROCEDURE 1:

The students are seated in a semicircle, facing the bulletin board. The teacher begins by holding up four cartoon drawings and asking the students to name the emotion depicted in each of the cartoons. Then he explains:

We have talked about our emotions. We have talked about our feelings. Today we are going to listen to four songs. Each song will tell how the singer feels. The emotion each singer feels is also the emotion found in one of the four cartoon faces. When you have told me how the singer feels, I will place the cartoon drawing of that same emotion on the bulletin board.

The students listen to the first song. When the song is finished, the teacher asks:

John, what was that person feeling when he sang his song to us?

John responds:

He was sad.

The teacher agrees and places the cartoon sad face on the bulletin board.

This activity continues until each student can verbally identify the four emotions.

MATERIALS: Typewritten copy of a song lyric for each student;
              two recordings of current songs; record player

PROCEDURE 2:   The students are seated in a semicircle. The teacher
                leads the class in a brief review of previous lessons
                which described the concept "emotions." He explains:

    We are going to listen to a song. See if you
    can identify what emotion the singer is ex-
    periencing.

The teacher plays the recording and the class listens. When
it is completed, the teacher asks:

    Jim, what do you think the singer felt as he
    sang that song?

Jim responds:

    He was frightened and sad.

The teacher replies:

    Good, Jim.

    I am going to give all of you a copy of that
    song.

When the song sheets have been distributed, the teacher reads
the words of the song to the class to be sure the students
understand the words. The teacher indicates:

    Each of us will change the words of the song.
    When we do this, we will change the "mood" or
    "feeling." Instead of a sad mood, we can
    change it to a happy, angry, lonely, excited
    or longing one.

When the teacher is certain the students understand the assignment, he allots time to complete the word changes. He is available to each student for suggestions or for help in spelling. When the students have completed the assignment, each student reads his lyrics aloud. The other class members verbally identify the mood or feeling depicted in each student's lyrics.

This activity continues until each student has had the opportunity to read his lyrics to the class and to identify the mood of another student's lyrics.

OBJECTIVE: Each Student Can Verbalize a Personal Experience in Which an Emotion Was Involved

MATERIALS: Chalk; chalkboard; eraser

PROCEDURE 1:

The students are seated at their desks, facing the chalkboard.
The teacher begins:

> Today we are going to talk about emotions.
> Let's see how many emotions we can name. As
> you name them, I will write them on the
> board.

After the students have named a number of emotions, which
the teacher has listed on the board, the teacher encourages
them to discuss the emotions listed on the board. The teacher
notes:

> We have talked about all the emotions listed
> on the board. The first emotion we discussed
> was anger. Raise your hand if you have ever
> been angry.

After those students who have experienced anger (all of them
should have) have raised their hands, the teacher continues:

> I see that most of the members of the class
> have been angry. Each of you may tell the

class who or what made you angry and what
you did when you became angry.

The teacher selects a student to share his experience with
the class. After the student has recalled his experience,
explaining the cause of the emotional reaction and the re-
sulting behavior, the teacher chooses another student to do
likewise.

This activity continues until each student has had a chance
to recall his emotional experience to the class.

MATERIALS: Chalk; chalkboard; eraser

PROCEDURE 2:

The students are seated in a semicircle, facing the chalk-board. The teacher begins:

> Today we are going to talk about feelings.
> Who can name a feeling that you have expe-
> rienced?

The teacher pauses and allows the students to name various feelings which they have experienced. After a number of feelings have been identified by the students, the teacher continues:

> Very good. You have named many feelings that
> you have experienced. Today I am going to
> ask you to think about the time when you ex-
> perienced a special feeling. I want you to
> share your experience with the class. I will
> write sentences on the board that will help
> you tell several different things in your
> story.

The teacher writes the following sentences on the board:

1. Where was I when the feeling happened?
2. Who was with me?
3. What made the feeling happen?
4. What did I do when the feeling happened?
5. Did I do the right thing?

After the teacher has written the sentences on the board and has read them to the class, he asks:

> Who has experienced anger?

The teacher then selects a volunteer to tell about experienc-ing anger. The teacher says:

33

Mary will tell about a time when she was
angry. She will answer the questions on the
board after I read them.

After Mary has shared her experience with the class, the
teacher instructs her to select a classmate to tell of his
personal experience with anger.

After the classmate has told of his experience, the teacher
introduces a new emotion, such as jealousy, and selects a
volunteer from the class to tell about a personal experience
with that emotion.

This activity continues until each student has had the opportunity to relate his personal experience with an emotion.

OBJECTIVE: Each Student Can Role Play a Story, Demonstrating Appropriate Emotional Responses to Given Situations

---

MATERIALS: Pictures which depict fear, anger, sadness, happiness

PROCEDURE 1:

The students are seated in a semicircle. The teacher has a series of pictures depicting situations in which the emotions fear, anger, sadness and happiness are represented.   The teacher remarks:

Today we are going to look at some pictures. These are pictures of people. These people have feelings just as you and I do. When we look at the pictures, we can tell how the people in the pictures are feeling.

The teacher selects one picture, displays it and continues:

Look at this picture. Who can tell us what is happening in it?

Then the teacher calls on volunteers to discuss the activity in the picture. After the class has discussed the situation in the picture, the teacher encourages the students to determine the feelings of the people in the picture. The teacher explains:

We have talked about the picture and we understand what the people are feeling. Now you

are going to be actors and actresses. You
are going to act out what is happening in the
picture.

After the teacher has selected volunteers to act out what is
depicted in the picture, he assists them in their presentation. Then he selects a second picture and explains:

Look at this picture. It tells a story. If
we look at the picture, we can tell what the
people in the picture are doing and how they
are feeling. There are two people in this
picture, a little girl and her mother.

Marie, what is the mother doing? How is she
feeling?

Betty, what is the little girl doing? How
is she feeling?

After Marie and Betty have verbalized the plot of the story
depicted in the picture and have demonstrated an understanding
of the emotional interaction, the teacher instructs them to
act out the story for the class.

The activity continues until each student has had an opportunity to act out a story and to express the emotions appropriate to the situation.

MATERIALS: Large jar containing several slips of paper, each of
which contains a written situation designed to elicit
an emotional response; chalk; chalkboard; eraser

PROCEDURE 2:

The students are seated at their desks, facing the chalkboard.
The teacher begins:

Today we are going to talk about emotions.
Emotions are feelings. All people have
feelings. Let's see how many feelings or
emotions you can name. I will write them
on the chalkboard.

After the students have named a number of emotions and the
teacher has listed them on the board, the teacher continues:

You have identified many emotions or feelings.
Listen as I name them.

After the students are familiar with the words, the teacher
explains:

On my desk is a jar. The jar contains several
slips of paper. On each slip is a story. The
stories tell of different situations that each
of you might experience. When I call your
name, select a slip of paper from the jar.
Read the story to the class. Choose classmates to help you act out the story. Before
you act out the story, think of how the
characters in the story are feeling. What
emotions will the characters demonstrate?
Be sure you understand and can show the
appropriate emotions while you are role playing the situation.

The teacher selects a volunteer to initiate the procedure.

This activity continues until each student can role play a story, demonstrating appropriate emotional responses to given situations.

Note: The stories might be composed of the following situations:

1. A teacher unfairly accuses a student of cheating.
2. A boy is rejected for a date.
3. A girl receives her first speeding ticket.
4. A purse is stolen from a girl's locker.
5. A favorite sister gives birth to twins.
6. A student is selected to serve as class president.

MATERIALS: Poster board; three signs on which the following words
             are printed, one on each sign: "Health," "Appearance,"
             "Behavior"; thumbtacks

PROCEDURE 1:

The students are seated in a semicircle. The teacher and
students discuss the word "responsibility." Through their
discussion, they arrive at the conclusion that "responsibility" means "taking care of one's self," "being accountable
for one's actions" and "being worthy of trust." The teacher
explains:

     I have responsibilities as a teacher. I must
     prepare lessons for you. I must be sure each
     of you understands our lessons.

     We all have responsibilities. I am going to
     put these three signs on our poster board.
     This one says "Health . . . How I Feel."
     This one says "Appearance . . . How I Look."
     The third one says "Behavior . . . How I
     Act."

After the teacher has put the three signs on the poster
board, he says:

     Now we are going to discuss what is printed on
     each of these three signs. First, in what
     ways can we be responsible for our health?

For each answer, I will put a thumbtack on
the sign.

The students are encouraged to respond with "be clean";
"don't smoke"; "get enough sleep"; "eat healthful food";
"use a toothbrush after every meal"; "lose excess weight";
"take a daily bath or shower."

The teacher puts a thumbtack on the sign for each response.
Then, he asks:

How many thumbtacks have we on the sign
"Health"? Yes, there are seven thumbtacks.
We know seven ways to be responsible for our
own health.

Now we will think of all the ways we can be
responsible for our appearance. How can we
be responsible for how we look?

Student responses might include "comb hair"; "wash and iron
clothes"; "use good posture"; "hang up our clothes"; "shine
our shoes."

Again, the teacher puts a thumbtack on the sign for each
response and then asks the students how many are on the sign
"Appearance."

Next, the teacher introduces the sign "Behavior" and then
asks how each student can be responsible for how he acts.

Answers might include the following responses: "be helpful
at home"; "be honest"; "obey traffic laws"; "be cheerful";
"obey school rules."

Once again, the teacher puts a thumbtack on the sign for
each response and then asks how many tacks are on the sign
"Behavior."

At the end of this activity, each student should have had an
opportunity to respond with a way he can be responsible in
"Health"; "Appearance"; or "Behavior."

Note: This activity may be reinforced by inviting individuals
       in responsible positions, such as a hair stylist, a
       nurse, a psychologist, etc., during the school term.
       These individuals not only would reinforce the sense

of responsibility but also would add new dimensions in vocabulary and experience.

<u>MATERIALS</u>: Newsprint; felt-tipped pen; oven timer

<u>PROCEDURE 2</u>:

The students are seated at their desks. The teacher introduces the word "responsibility" to the students and discusses
the meaning of the word with them. Then he arranges the
students in small groups and explains:

> I will set our timer for 10 minutes. During
> this time, each group should choose a leader
> who will lead his particular group in a dis-
> cussion of the various areas in which we
> should demonstrate responsible behavior. At
> the end of the 10-minute period, each group
> leader will report to the class what his group
> has determined to be areas in which we should
> exercise responsible behavior.

The groups work independently of each other until the timer
signals an end to group discussion. Each leader reports his
group's responses to the class, and the teacher records them
on the newsprint. (Example areas could include hygiene,
work, appearance.) Next, the teacher explains:

> Each of you will select one of the responsi-
> bility areas from the recorded list. (There
> can be no more than two class members per
> area.) I will record your name and responsi-
> bility area so that the other class members
> will know which one you have chosen. Then
> you may tell the class ways that you can be
> responsible in everyday life in this parti-
> cular area.

This activity continues until each student has had an opportunity to tell the class how he can be responsible in the
area he has selected.

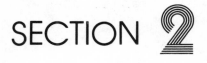

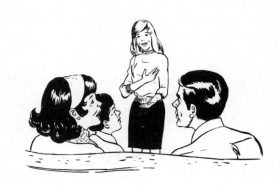

I Am a Family Member

The authors recognize that in today's society, there are many students who do not have a "family" in the traditional sense of the word; nevertheless, all students have some type of surrogate family relationship.

The authors have provided notes at the end of the lesson plans which explain in detail how to accomplish the objectives with students who are living in a center or in a foster home.

For the students whose parents are divorced, the concept of step-relationships should be introduced in the same manner as immediate family relationships.

OBJECTIVE: Each Student Can Demonstrate an Understanding of the Concept, "Family"

MATERIALS: Paper; pencils; chalk; chalkboard; eraser

PROCEDURE 1:

The students are seated at their desks, facing the chalkboard. The teacher writes the word "family" on the chalkboard and explains:

> Today you are going to learn what the word
> "family" means. We often use the word. Mary
> has told us that her family is coming to our
> open house. Yesterday I said that I did not
> know that John had two brothers in his family.

The teacher directs the discussion so that the students are able to volunteer ideas such as "a family may be people who live under one roof"; "a family may be people who are related"; "a family may be people who have a common history." When the teacher is certain that each student has an understanding of the concept, the students are directed to draw a picture of where their family lives.

When the pictures are completed, the teacher remarks:

> John Burke, you may show us your picture.
> John's family lives in a mobile home. I will
> write "Burke family" on your picture, John.
> Please tell us about your family.

John responds:

> My family has five people: my mother, my two
> brothers, my sister and me. My family came
> from Texas. My father lives in Texas. He
> did not move here with us. My family likes it
> here. We like our mobile home on Oak Street.

The teacher comments:

> Good, John, you have told us many things about
> your family. I will write the number 5 under
> your Burke family picture, as you have five
> people in your family.

This activity continues until each student is able to demonstrate an understanding of the concept, "family."

Note: Prior to this activity, the teacher should ask those
students who have no immediate families if they wish
to discuss their lifestyles with their classmates.
For those students who agree to do so, the teacher
asks each of them to draw a picture of his home.

During the activity, the teacher explains:

> Terry lives in a home that is different
> from most of yours. He lives at
> Milltown Center. He would like to
> tell us about the people at the center
> who are his family. Although Terry is
> not related to the people at the
> center, in many ways these people are
> his family.
>
> Terry, please tell us about the people
> at the center who are special to you.

Those students who live in foster homes may follow
the procedure in a manner similar to the one just
mentioned.

46

MATERIALS: Name labels, one for each student; pictures of many
              types of houses--igloo, fantasy space house, farm,
              ranch, castle; bulletin board; thumbtacks

PROCEDURE 2:

The students are seated in a semicircle, facing the bulletin
board. The teacher initiates a discussion of the concept,
"family." The discussions should encompass the following
ideas: "family members usually share a common dwelling";
"family members are related to one another"; "family members
share a common history."

The teacher places the pictures of the houses on the bulletin
board and distributes a label to each student. Then, he
explains:

      Write your last name and the word "family" on
      your label. Think of the many things that
      you know about your family. When you can
      tell five facts about your family, using com-
      plete sentences, you may place your label on
      one of the house pictures which are on the
      bulletin board.

      Ann, you may begin.

Ann responds:

      My family has four people in it: my mother,
      father, sister and me. My sister and I were
      born here, but my father was born in Puerto
      Rico, and my mother was born in Florida. We
      have lived on Tyson Street since I was born.

      Everyone in my family is away during the day.
      My mother and father work, my sister and I go
      to school. But we like to eat dinner together,
      and we tell each other what happened during
      the day.

The teacher comments:

Excellent, Ann. You know many things about
your family. You may choose a picture from
the bulletin board. Place your name label
on the picture.

This activity continues until each student can demonstrate
an understanding of the concept, "family."

Note: If some students have no immediate families, the
teacher should ask them, prior to this activity, if
they wish to discuss the special people, such as
foster parents or cottage parents, who act as family
members. For those students who agree to do so,
during the activity each of them should be given a
label with his surname written on it. The teacher
remarks:

Mary lives with her foster parents,
Mr. and Mrs. Smith. Mary is not related to the Smiths, but they are her
substitute parents. Mary will tell
us five facts about the family she
lives with.

Those students who live in centers or in group homes
may discuss special people in their centers or homes.

MATERIALS: Pictures of families, one picture for each student;
             one large picture of a family

PROCEDURE 1:

The students are seated in a semicircle. The teacher holds
up a large picture of a family, visible to all students.
The teacher explains:

    You have learned many things about the word
    "family." Here is a picture of a family.
    Let's make up a name for the family in this
    picture. Let's call the family the Jones
    family.

    Bob, point to Mrs. Jones. Good. Why did you
    point to her? Yes, she is older. She must
    be the mother.

    Pat, point to Mr. Jones. Fine. Why did you
    point to him? Yes, he is older. He must be
    the father.

    Ed, point to the daughters. Very good. Why
    did you point to them? Yes, they are all
    girls, and they are all younger than the
    mother. They must be the daughters.

    John, point to the sons. Well done. Why
    did you point to them? Yes, they are all
    boys, and they are all younger than the
    father. They must be the sons.

The teacher continues this activity until each student can identify the various family members in the picture. Then, he repeats the procedure, using a different picture for each student.

This activity continues until each student has had an opportunity to identify all family members in his picture.

MATERIALS: Eight pictures of families from different parts of
             the world; bulletin board; thumbtacks

PROCEDURE 2:

The students are seated in a semicircle, facing the bulletin
board. The teacher places the pictures of families from
different parts of the world on the bulletin board in view
of the students. The teacher explains:

> Look at these eight pictures I have tacked to
> our bulletin board. Each picture shows a
> family. Each family lives in a different
> part of the world. In every picture, we see
> the mother, father, grandmother (s), grand-
> father (s), son (s) and daughter (s).

Then the teacher continues:

> Tom, you may point to the daughters in each
> of the eight pictures.

When Tom has done this, the teacher asks the students why
Tom selected the girls in the pictures. Responses should
include "daughters are girls" and "they are younger than the
mother and grandmother."

As the lesson continues, the teacher may introduce more com-
plicated concepts; for example, he may have the students
point to the son of the grandfather in each picture or point
to the oldest family member in each picture.

This activity continues until each student can identify
family members in pictures.

MATERIALS: Flannel board; figures of a mother, father, teenage
boy, teenage girl; string; chalk; chalkboard; eraser

PROCEDURE 1:

The students are seated at their desks, facing the chalkboard. The teacher writes the words "immediate family" on
the board and explains:

We have talked about the word "family." You
have heard the expression "immediate family."
Today you are going to learn what "immediate
family" means. Look at the flannel board.
Here is a mother. Here is a father. They
have two children, a boy and a girl. They
are an immediate family. They make a family.

Watch as I encircle our family with string.
In the circle is an immediate family.
Immediate means there is nothing between the
circle and the family. Nothing outside that
circle can come into that family. We could
put a line to the mother's mother. We know
this would be the grandmother, but the grandmother is outside the circle. Only the
mother, father and children make up an immediate family.

I will draw a big circle on the chalkboard.
Inside the circle I will put the names of
John's immediate family.

John, you may tell us who is in your family.
I will write their names on the board.

53

John responds:

My mother, father, sisters and brothers. My
sisters' names are Pat, Aggie and Mozelle.
My brothers' names are Tony, George and Pete.

The teacher replies:

Good, John. Now, we know the names of the
members of your immediate family. How many
sons do your mom and dad have?

John answers:

They have four.

The teacher asks:

How many brothers do you have?

John answers:

I have three brothers.

The teacher replies:

That is correct. How many sisters do you
have?

John answers:

I have three sisters.

The teacher remarks:

John knows who the members of his immediate family are.

This activity continues until each student can identify immediate family relationships.

Note: Those students who do not have immediate families may also be included in this activity. They may identify the members of immediate families in sample pictures. They may also answer the following questions regarding each sample picture of an immediate family:

   1. What family members make up the immediate family?
   2. How many sons are in the immediate family?
   3. How many daughters are in the immediate family?

MATERIALS: Copies of local newspapers, with obituary and birth
           announcement sections, one for each student; chalk;
           chalkboard; eraser

PROCEDURE 2:

The students are seated in a semicircle, facing the chalkboard. The teacher remarks:

> Last night I went to visit a friend in the
> hospital. I went to the desk and asked if I
> could see Paula Sullivan. The lady at the
> desk said, "I'm sorry, Mrs. Sullivan can only
> have her immediate family visit her." What
> do you suppose that lady meant by "immediate
> family"? Who is in your "immediate family"?

The teacher writes the correct responses on the board. When
the responses have included "mother," "father," "sons,"
"daughters," "brothers," "sisters," the teacher explains:

> Many times we see the words "immediate family"
> in the paper. I brought each of you a copy of
> the newspaper because I saw the words "immedi-
> ate family" used over and over again. They
> were used on page 7.
>
> John, please give everyone his own copy of the
> paper.
>
> When you get your paper, turn to page 7.

When all the students have turned to page 7, the teacher
continues:

> Look at the word "obituary." It comes from
> an old word meaning "to go to meet," "to die."
> The obituary page is a page found in the news-
> paper. Names of people who have died recently
> are printed on the obituary page. Look at the
> first name in the obituary column. The first
> name is "Flanagan, James, 62." The "62" tells
> the age of Mr. Flanagan. The article also

says: "Funeral services for immediate family only."

Who do you think can come to the funeral, John?

John responds:

His children and his wife.

The teacher agrees:

Good, John. Only his children and wife are to go to the funeral. They are his immediate family. Now let's look at the announcement section. It is right across from the obituaries. "Announcement" comes from an old word meaning "to tell the news."

These are birth announcements. These tell about babies who were born yesterday. Let's look at the first one. I will read it:

Mr. and Mrs. George Waters, 17298 South Central Ave., a girl, 8 pounds, 13½ ounces, or 4 kilograms, 12:58 a.m., Nov. 8.

The 8 pounds, 13½ ounces, or 4 kilograms, tells us how much Mr. and Mrs. George Waters' baby weighed when she was born. There is something about this little baby girl we don't know from this announcement. What don't we know, Mary?

Mary thinks and responds:

We don't know her name.

The teacher replies:

57

Well done, Mary. We do not know her immediate
family either. Let's make up an immediate
family for her.

John, who else can be in her immediate family?

John responds:

Her brothers and sisters.

The teacher comments:

Good, John. Her mother, father, brothers and
sisters are her immediate family.

Now that we are sure that we know what "immediate family" means, I want each of you to
tell us who is in your immediate family.

Each student tells the class the members of his immediate
family. The teacher writes the names on the board.

This activity continues until each student can identify his
immediate family relationships.

Note: Those students who do not have immediate families may
identify immediate family relationships by answering
questions about the obituary and birth announcement
exercises, as has been demonstrated in this activity.

```
┌─────────────────────────────────────────────────────────────────┐
│ OBJECTIVE: Each Student Can Non-verbally Identify Extended Family Relation- │
│            ships Represented in Pictures                          │
└─────────────────────────────────────────────────────────────────┘
```

MATERIALS: Pictures of one student's grandparents, maternal and
              paternal; pictures of the same student's aunts and
              uncles; pictures of grandmothers, grandfathers, aunts
              and uncles of each student; overhead projector;
              bulletin board; thumbtacks

PROCEDURE 1:

    (Prior to this activity, the teacher has collected from the
    family of each class member pictures of the following rela-
    tives: grandmothers, grandfathers, aunts, uncles, and has
    placed these pictures in rows across the bulletin board.)

    The students are seated in a semicircle, facing the projector.
    The teacher begins:

        Today we are going to talk about members of
        Terri's family. All the people in the family
        are related--that is why they are called rela-
        tives. I will point to the family members
        and tell who they are. Listen carefully.

    The teacher points to each picture, identifying the people
    in the pictures as grandmothers, grandfathers, aunts, uncles.
    The teacher explains:

        The relatives we will discuss today are part
        of an extended family. They are not part of
        an immediate family. Remember, immediate
        family members include mother, father, sisters

59

and brothers. All other relatives are part
of an extended family. Grandmothers, grandfathers, aunts and uncles are members of extended families.

Terri has many relatives. She has two grandmothers, two grandfathers, two aunts, one
uncle. Let's talk about Terri's grandmothers
first. I will put the pictures of Terri's
grandmothers on the projector. We will see
the pictures on the wall.

The teacher places the pictures of the two grandmothers on
the overhead projector. He points to each picture as he
identifies each of the grandmothers. He explains:

This is Grandmother Jones. She is Terri's
father's mother. She is Terri's grandmother.

The teacher then points to the picture of Terri's other
grandmother and explains:

This is Grandmother Brown. She is Terri's
mother's mother. She is Terri's grandmother,
also. Terri has two grandmothers who are
both living.

The teacher removes the pictures of the grandmothers, places
the pictures of the student's grandfathers on the overhead
projector and identifies them in the same manner.

After the teacher has identified the grandfathers and grandmothers, he places the pictures of the student's two aunts
on the overhead projector and identifies them by saying:

These are Terri's aunts. This is Aunt Lucille,
and this is Aunt Marie. Aunt Lucille is
Terri's father's sister. Aunt Marie is the
sister of Terri's mother. Both of Terri's
aunts are the children of Terri's grandparents.

After the aunts have been identified, the teacher identifies
Terri's uncle in a similar manner. The teacher explains:

60

This is Terri's uncle. He is the brother of
Terri's father. He is a child of Terri's
Grandmother and Grandfather Jones. Terri
has only one uncle.

After all of Terri's relatives have been identified, the
teacher continues:

Now let's see if you can find the relatives I
have been talking about. I will place the
pictures on the bulletin board.

After the teacher has placed the pictures on the bulletin
board, he says:

Larry, please come to the board. Find Terri's
mother's mother.

If Larry cannot point to the picture, the teacher says:

Watch while I point to the picture of Terri's
mother's mother. We also call this person
Terri's grandmother.

Now point to the picture of Terri's mother's
mother.

If Larry can point to the picture, the teacher adds:

Yes, that is Terri's mother's mother. We can
also say she is Terri's grandmother. Can you
find Terri's father's mother? She is also
Terri's grandmother.

After Larry has identified Terri's grandmothers, this activity
continues until all the family members' pictures on the board
have been identified by Terri's classmates.

Note: The teacher should encourage each student to bring to
class pictures of aunts, uncles, grandmothers and
grandfathers. Each student's family relationships
should be discussed in class.

MATERIALS: Pictures of grandmothers, grandfathers, aunts, uncles,
             cousins, nephews and nieces of one student; overhead
             projector; bulletin board; thumbtacks

PROCEDURE 2:

The students are seated at their desks, facing the projector
and the bulletin board. The teacher places the pictures of
the student's cousin on the overhead projector and explains:

    Now we see a picture of Betty's cousin. Cousins
    are children of aunts and uncles. This is
    Betty's cousin, William. He is the child of
    Aunt Lucille and Uncle Louis.

After the teacher has introduced Betty's cousin, he removes
the picture of the cousin and places pictures of Betty's
nephews on the projector and continues:

    Here are pictures of Betty's nephews. She has
    two nephews. Their names are Ted and John.
    Ted is Betty's brother's son. John is Betty's
    sister's son. They are both Betty's nephews.

The teacher removes the pictures of Betty's nephews and puts
a picture of Betty's niece on the projector. The teacher
continues:

    This is Betty's niece. Her name is Jane.
    She is Betty's brother's child.

The teacher removes the picture from the projector and places
all the relatives' pictures on the bulletin board. The
teacher explains:

    We have talked about the people in the pictures
    on the bulletin board. They are all Betty's
    relatives.

62

Jerry, please come to the board and point to
Betty's aunt and uncle's child. He is Betty's
cousin.

After Jerry has identified Betty's cousin, the teacher
instructs:

Jerry, now find the picture of Betty's niece.
She is Betty's brother's child.

This activity continues until each student can identify extended family relationships represented in the pictures.

Note: This procedure is identical to Procedure 1, except
that the extended family relationships of cousin,
niece and nephew are also introduced. As in Procedure 1, the teacher should introduce the relatives
of one student's grandmothers, grandfathers, aunts
and uncles.

OBJECTIVE: Each Student Can Describe a Family Member

MATERIALS: Pictures of students' families in informal situations;
oaktag paper; full-length mirror; bulletin board;
thumbtacks

PROCEDURE 1:

(Prior to this activity, the teacher has collected candid
photos of family members from students' families. These
photos have been taped to a large piece of oaktag paper, and
the paper has been affixed to the bulletin board. A full-
length mirror has been placed beside the bulletin board.)

The students are seated in a semicircle, facing the bulletin
board. The teacher directs the students' attention to the
mirror and explains:

Today you are going to describe yourselves and
the immediate members of your families.
"Describe," as you recall, means "to tell how
someone or something looks."

Patty, you may stand in front of the mirror.
Please tell the class how you look.

After Patty has finished her description, the teacher praises
her and then calls upon members of the class to contribute
additional descriptive words. The teacher adds:

You have told us many words that describe yourself, Patty. You may go to the pictures on the
bulletin board and find a member of your
family. Don't tell us whom you have chosen.

When Patty is ready, the teacher explains:

> You may describe the family member you have
> chosen. Use as many descriptive words as you
> can. Try to give us a picture by using these
> words. When you are finished, we will select
> one of the students to come to the board and
> try to find the person you have described.

After Patty has completed her description, the teacher chooses
a student to identify the person Patty has described.

This activity continues until each student has had the opportunity to describe himself and a family member.

<u>Note</u>: Those students who have no immediate families should
be asked to describe the people with whom they live.

MATERIALS: Pictures of students' families; overhead projector;
            red chips

PROCEDURE 2:

The students are seated at their desks, facing the projector.
The teacher explains:

> I have a picture of John's family to show you
> on our projector. Look at John's mother. Who
> can describe her to us so that we will know
> this is John's mother? For every sentence you
> use to describe her, I will give you one red
> chip. Let us see who can earn 10 chips.
>
> Mary, you may begin.

Mary might say:

> John's mother is a pretty lady. She is tall
> and thin. She wears glasses. She has blond
> hair. She looks like a happy person.

The teacher praises her:

> Good, Mary, you have described John's mother
> to us. You have earned five chips.

After all the family members in all the pictures have been
identified and described by the students, the teacher
explains:

> Now I will give each of you the picture of
> your own family members. You have heard your
> classmates describe members of your family.
> Perhaps you will be able to add to the de-
> scriptions they have given.

Tonya, you may begin. Tell us which member
of your family you will describe. Bring that
person's photo to me.

The teacher identifies the person in the photo, tells his
relationship to the student and places the picture on the
projector. The teacher explains:

Tonya will describe her father for us. Remember, "to describe" means "to tell about."
Tonya may tell us things about her father
that we cannot see in the photo, as well as
things we can see in the photo.

This activity continues until each student has had the opportunity to describe a family member, thus earning up to
10 chips.

Note: The teacher should follow the same course of action
       as described in the note of Procedure 1.

MATERIALS: Pictures of a mother and father, two grandmothers, two grandfathers, an aunt and an uncle; bulletin board; thumbtacks

PROCEDURE 1:

(Prior to this activity, the family relationships of mother, father, grandmother and grandfather, aunt and uncle were introduced, and each student was able to identify these family members nonverbally.)

The students are seated in a semicircle, facing the bulletin board. The teacher assembles pictures of two grandmothers, two grandfathers, a mother and a father, an aunt and an uncle and places them on the bulletin board. Then, the teacher explains:

> We have talked about these family members on the board. Listen carefully as I point to them and tell who they are.

The teacher points to the picture of a grandmother and explains:

> This is a grandmother. She is mother's mother. I will put the picture of this grandmother beside our picture of mother.

> This is a picture of a grandmother also. There are two grandmothers on the board. This is father's mother. We will put the picture of this grandmother beside the picture of father.

69

This is an aunt. An aunt may be mother's or
father's sister. This aunt is mother's
sister. We will put her picture beside
mother's picture.

This is an uncle. An uncle may be mother's
or father's brother. This uncle is father's
brother. I will put the picture of the uncle
beside father's picture.

Now listen carefully. I will point to all
the pictures and explain who the people are.
Then I will ask you to identify the people
in the pictures, in terms of their family
relationship to each other.

The teacher points to each picture and, after telling who
each family member is again, explains the family relationship. Then he continues:

Each of you may now identify the people in
the pictures as to their family relationship.

John, you may begin. Please point to and
identify each family member.

If John is unable to identify each of the family members in
the pictures, the teacher points to each picture again and
names each family member again, explaining the family relationships.

I would like you to try to identify the people
in the pictures as to their family relationships. If you have difficulty, I will help
you once again.

If John is able to identify each of the family members in
the pictures, the teacher explains the family relationships
once again:

Yes, John, this is a grandmother. She is
father's mother.

The teacher continues:

You may answer some questions about family members. We will see if you understand how the people in the family are related to one another.

Tom, who is father's mother? What do we call her?

If Tom is unable to identify the family members correctly, the teacher says:

Tom, this is the picture of father's mother. We call her grandmother. Now point to the picture of father's mother. What do we call her?

If Tom is able to answer the question correctly, the teacher comments:

Yes, Tom, father's mother is called grandmother. Very good.

This activity continues until each student has had the opportunity to identify family members and their relationships through verbal interaction with the teacher.

MATERIALS: Large oaktag cards, each bearing a word denoting a
              particular family member's relationship; chalk;
              chalkboard; eraser

PROCEDURE 2:

The students are seated at their desks, facing the chalkboard. The teacher provides each student with a large oaktag
card on which is written the name of a particular family
member's relationship. The teacher explains:

    Today we are going to talk about family rela-
    tionships. I will write the names of the
    various family members' relationships on the
    board.

After the teacher has written the words on the board, he
explains:

    Please listen as I read these. Each of you
    has one of these words written on the card
    on your desk.

The teacher then reads the words to the class. When he has
finished, he comments:

    You may look at your cards. What is the name
    of the family relationship which is written
    on your card?

The teacher has each student read the name of the family
member's relationship which is written on his card. If the
student is unable to identify the word, the teacher reads
it for the student, has the student match it to the word on
the board and has the student say it aloud.

Once all the cards have been identified, the teacher continues:

    I will tell you about one of the family mem-
    ber's relationships. When I tell you about

this family member whose name is written on
your card, raise your hand and identify the
name of the family relationship.

After the teacher has given instructions to the students, he
points to the first word on the board and tells the family
member's relationship. The teacher asks:

What do we call the man who is mother's
brother? Who has the word that will tell
this?

If the student who has the word "uncle" raises his hand and
identifies the word, the teacher praises him and collects
his card.

When each student has identified the relationship on the
card which he holds, identifying the family member who fits
the teacher's description, the teacher redistributes the
cards to the class. This activity continues until each
student can identify all family members' relationships by
name.

Note: The ability to identify the family relationships of
       mother, father, sister, brother, daughter, son, grand-
       mother, grandfather, aunt, uncle, niece, nephew,
       cousin, nonverbally, is a prerequisite for this
       activity.

OBJECTIVE: Each Student Can Express Family Relationships in Sentences

MATERIALS: Full-face masks to represent family members (may be made of poster board and mounted on popsicle sticks)

PROCEDURE 1:

(Prior to this activity, the teacher has made full-face masks to represent family members discussed in this lesson. These masks may be made from poster board and mounted on popsicle sticks, which should serve as handles for the masks.)

The students are seated at their desks. The teacher begins:

Today we are going to talk about family. Some of you will wear a family member mask.

The teacher directs a student to come to the front of the class and gives the following instructions:

Harold, you may be the brother in the family. A brother is mother and father's son. Here is the brother's mask. Stand in front of the class and hold the mask to your face. Remember, a brother is mother and father's son.

The teacher assigns roles until each family member is represented and gives each student who represents a family member a mask to wear. After he has assigned the roles and given out the masks, he explains:

All the family members have been chosen.
Those students who are seated will pretend
that they do not know our family members.
They will go to each family member and say,
"Who are you?" Each family member will tell
who he is and how he is related to another
family member.

Charlene, you may help me show the class what
to do. Come to the front of the class and
choose a family member. Ask the family member
the question, "Who are you?"

After Charlene has asked one of the family members the
question, the teacher comments:

Good, Charlene. You have asked Marie who she
is. Now Marie will tell us in a sentence who
she is.

If Marie responds, "I am the mother," the teacher replies:

Fine, Marie. Now tell us how you are related
to someone else in the family. Remember to
use a sentence.

If Marie is unable to do so, the teacher offers help in
identifying the family relationship, by saying:

Marie is the mother. She is father's wife.
Marie, say: "I am father's wife."

After Marie has patterned the sentence, the teacher explains:

Marie is also Grandmother and Grandfather
Jones' daughter.

Marie may also say:

I am Grandmother and Grandfather Jones'
daughter.

The teacher continues to aid the students in expressing the characters' family relationships and in providing sentences for the students to pattern.

This activity continues until each student is able to express family relationships in sentence form.

<u>Note</u>: The degree and complexity of the relationships introduced by the teacher will depend on the ability and language level of the students.

MATERIALS: Oaktag cards, on which are printed the names of
              family members' relationships, one name per card;
              chalk; chalkboard; eraser

PROCEDURE 2:

The students are seated at their desks, facing the chalkboard. The teacher explains:

    Today we are going to talk about family rela-
    tionships. I will write the names of the
    family members' relationships on the board.

After the teacher has written the words on the board, he
explains:

    Listen as I read the words to you. When you
    know what the words are, I will give you a
    card with the name of one of the family mem-
    bers written on it. Look at the word and
    then turn the card over so that no one else
    can read it.

    If you cannot read the word, I will tell you
    what it is. Then you may tell us about the
    family member whose name is written on your
    card. Remember, do not tell the name; but,
    do tell about the person.

    Also, remember to use sentences. For example,
    if I had the word "niece," I might say:

        I am a girl. I am your brother's
        child. Who am I?

The teacher selects a volunteer to answer the question. If
the student answers correctly, but not in sentence form, the
teacher remarks:

    Your answer is correct, but you must remember
    to use sentences when answering the question.
    Give your answer this way: "You are a niece."

78

This activity continues until each student has had the opportunity to explain family relationships in sentence form.

OBJECTIVE: Each Student Can Complete a Story Involving a Family

MATERIALS: Sequenced action pictures involving family members; books made of construction paper, one book for each student

PROCEDURE 1:

(Prior to this activity, the teacher has collected sequenced action pictures involving family members. [These may be purchased commercially or collected from books or comic strips.] These sequenced action pictures have been pasted on construction paper to form the pages of a book. There is one book for each student.)

The students are seated in a semicircle. The teacher explains:

> Today you are going to help me tell stories about family members. Each of you will be given your own book. I will begin the story-telling for you. I want you to finish the story.

> Bill, you may go to the table and choose a book that you would like to share with the class.

After Bill has chosen a book, the teacher continues:

> Bill and I will be telling you a story about a family who is going on a trip. Look at the pictures as I begin the story. Bill, you may finish the story for us.

The teacher then holds the picture book in view of the
students and begins telling about the first two pictures in
the book. When the teacher finishes telling about the first
two pictures in the book, he encourages Bill to complete the
story for the class. The teacher says:

> I have told part of the story. Bill, what
> happens next? Please finish the story.

This activity continues until each student can complete a
story involving family interaction.

MATERIALS: Comic strips involving family activities, one comic
            strip for each class member; overhead projector

PROCEDURE 2:

(Prior to this activity, the teacher has brought to class
comic strips from the local newspaper, one comic strip for
each student.)

The students are seated at their desks, facing the projector.
The teacher asks:

    How many of you read the comics in the news-
    paper?

After the students have responded, the teacher asks them to
name their favorite comic strips. Then the teacher and
students discuss why a particular comic character is appeal-
ing. After the discussion, the teacher continues:

    Today we are going to tell stories about
    families. These are "special" families. They
    are the characters we see in the comic strips
    in our newspaper.

    I will begin the first story by telling what
    is happening in the first picture. I will
    then choose one of you to finish the story
    for the class. Then, we will go on to the
    next story, and so on.

    Before I begin each story, I will point to
    the characters and then name them to be sure
    that they are familiar to you. Let's begin.

This activity continues until each student has had several
opportunities to complete stories about comic strip families.

Note: After all the stories have been completed, the
       teacher may wish to lead the students into other
       discussions regarding how and when were the charac-
       ters in the various comics developed; what are the
       types of humor represented in different stories; what
       are some personal humorous family incidents which

might be portrayed in comic strip form. The students might enjoy drawing and narrating personal family incidents using this medium.

MATERIALS: Magazines and pairs of scissors, one of each for each
student

PROCEDURE 1:

(Prior to this activity, the teacher has collected an assort-
ment of magazines and pairs of scissors and has placed one
of each of these on each student's desk.)

The students are seated at their desks. The teacher begins:

> On your desks you will find a magazine and a
> pair of scissors. Look through the magazine
> and find three pictures of family members
> doing something together. They may be eat-
> ing, playing, riding in the car or perhaps
> talking. Cut the pictures out and place
> them on your desk. Put the magazine in your
> desk when you are finished.

After each student has placed the pictures on his desk and
put the magazine in his desk, the teacher gives the following
directions:

> Each of you has chosen three pictures. Look
> at the pictures. The family members are
> probably doing something that you have done
> with your families. Do the pictures remind
> you of something you like to do with your
> families? I want you to think of stories

about your own families and to share the
stories with the class.

Mary Lou, you may begin. Please bring your
picture to me. Which picture reminds you of
a story about your own family? You may tell
the story to the class.

After Mary Lou has selected a picture, the teacher places
the picture on the overhead projector and reflects the image
on the wall or on a screen for the rest of the class to view.
The teacher remarks:

Mary Lou has chosen a picture showing a family
on a picnic. She will tell us about her own
family going on a picnic.

The teacher formulates structure for the story by suggesting
information that might be included in the story. The teacher
says:

Mary Lou might tell us where they went, what
they did and what they ate. Mary Lou, you may
begin your story.

After Mary Lou has completed her story, the teacher selects
another student to tell a personal family story.

This activity continues until each student has had an opportunity to tell a story about his family members doing
something together.

Note: If some students are not living with their immediate
families, the teacher may vary the activity as
follows:

Don lives at Milltow Center. He is
not living with a family, but he will
tell about his cottage parents at the
center. He will tell of a special
activity that he and his cottage
parents have taken part in.

86

MATERIALS: Chalk; chalkboard; eraser

PROCEDURE 2:

The students are seated at their desks, facing the chalkboard. The teacher begins the activity by explaining:

> Today you are going to tell stories about your
> families. I'm sure that each of you will have
> an interesting story to tell. You will tell
> your stories in a special way. First, I will
> write some sentences on the board.

The teacher writes the following sentences on the board:

1.   Who is in the story?
2.   What are the people doing?
3.   What happened?
4.   What special feelings do I have about the
     story?

The teacher reads the sentences to the students, instructing
them to use the sentences as a guideline for storytelling.
The teacher continues:

> I will choose someone to begin a story. All of
> you must listen very carefully. After each
> story is told, I will choose a student to
> answer the questions on the board. Remember
> to listen very carefully.

The teacher then selects a student to begin the activity.
After the first student has finished his story, by following
the teacher's guidelines, the teacher generates spontaneous
storytelling about the family in the following manner:

> Larry has just finished his story about a
> family trip to Disney World. It was a very
> interesting story, and you were a good
> audience. Now I would like Lynn to answer
> the questions on the board.

If Lynn is unable to answer the questions on the board, the teacher says:

> Lynn needs the help of a good listener. Who
> can answer the questions on the board?

The teacher selects a volunteer to answer the questions.
After the volunteer has answered the questions, the teacher
says:

> Lynn, I will read the questions to you now. I
> would like you to answer the questions. I will
> call on you later to answer questions about
> another story.

After Lynn has answered the four questions on the board, the
teacher encourages other students to share stories about
special trips taken with their families. The teacher says:

> Perhaps some of you have also taken special
> family trips. Who, besides Larry, has a
> special trip to tell about?

When listening to the students' stories, the teacher may
find it necessary to remind students to provide all the information included in the sentence guidelines on the board.

This activity continues until each student has had the opportunity to tell a story about an activity shared by all
his family members.

Note: Those students who have no immediate families may
       tell a story about foster parents, cottage parents
       or counselors, as in the note of Procedure 1.

MATERIALS: Picture of a mother and a father; chalk; chalkboard; eraser

PROCEDURE 1:

The students are seated at their desks, facing the chalk-board. The teacher begins:

Today we are going to talk about a very important word. The word is "responsibility." A responsible person, as you may remember, is one who has a job to do and does it the very best he can. The responsible person knows that he should take care of himself and others as best he can. The responsible person takes care of his belongings in the best way possible.

I am going to tell you about a boy named Ray. He is a responsible person. I will tell you some of the ways that Ray is a responsible person and a responsible family member. Listen as I tell about Ray.

At home, Ray has jobs to do. He does each job as best he can. He is cheerful as he works.

At home, Ray is courteous and kind to the members of his family. He is responsible for helping to keep his home a happy place in which to live.

At home, Ray keeps his belongings in his room.
He is responsible for helping to keep the
house neat and in order.

At home, Ray keeps medicine he must take in
the medicine cabinet out of the reach of
little children. He is responsible for
keeping his brothers and sisters safe.

These are some of Ray's responsibilities at
home. Perhaps you can think of other responsibilities that Ray may have at home.
Just like Ray, you have responsibilities at
home also. Think of them now. I will write
all of them on the board. When you can tell
us about a responsibility you have at home,
raise your hand.

The teacher pauses, giving students an opportunity to think
of home responsibilities. After a number of students have
volunteered, the teacher calls on each student and writes
the responsibilities on the board.

After each student has contributed at least one responsibility, the teacher remarks:

You have done a very good job of telling me
your responsibilities as a family member. Now
I will put a picture of mother and father on
our board. They have responsibilities also.
As you tell their responsibilities, I will
write them on the board. We will begin with
mother's responsibilities. Who would like to
begin?

This activity continues until each student is able to demonstrate an understanding of the concept, "responsibility,"
and is able to define responsibilities that he and others
must have in regard to family life.

Note: For those students who are not living with their
        immediate families, the teacher may rephrase direc-
        tions, as in the following example:

        Tony, you live in a special kind of
        home. What are some of your responsi-
        bilities in the home in which you live?

90

What responsibilities do you have to
the other people who live in your
special home?

MATERIALS: Art supplies for making posters (these might include
              rubber cement or glue, scissors, poster board, rulers,
              packages of multi-colored construction paper, boxes
              of crayons or colored pencils); magazines; long table;
              chalk; chalkboard; eraser

PROCEDURE 2:

(Prior to this activity, the teacher has gathered up art
supplies and magazines to be used by the students in making
their posters. These materials have been placed on the table
in the back of the room.)

The students are seated at their desks, facing the chalkboard. The teacher begins:

Today we are going to talk about responsibility. Everyone has responsibilities.
Before we begin talking about responsibilities, we need to know what "responsibility"
means. We will say that we are going "to
define responsibility." When we define a
word, we tell what it means. We could use
a dictionary, a book of words, to tell us
what responsibility means. Let's see if
you can tell what the word means.

The teacher then guides the students in defining "responsibility." The teacher may wish to offer a simplified version
of the dictionary definition after the students have at-
tempted spontaneous definitions.

Once the word has been defined, the teacher continues:

Everyone has responsibilities. I will name
some people who do. You may tell some responsibilities that those people probably
have.

The teacher names members of various occupations, such as
doctors, policemen, bankers, teachers, bus drivers, and instructs the students to tell of responsibilities associated
with those people's jobs.

92

After students have demonstrated an understanding of the responsibilities of the people named, the activity focuses on the individual responsibilities of the students as family members. The teacher explains:

> Each of you has responsibilities. Today we will talk about your responsibilities as a family member. Each of you will tell at least one responsibility you have as a family member. I am going to write them on the board as you name them.

The teacher gives each student an opportunity to contribute ideas to the class discussion and lists them on the board.

After the students have demonstrated an understanding of the concept, "responsibility," in regard to family life, the teacher remarks:

> I have written many responsibilities of family life on the board. They are all important in making family life successful. I think we should show other members of the school just how important it is to be a responsible family member and to show many ways in which we can be responsible family members. Each of you will make a poster showing one of the responsibilities we have discussed and written on the board. You may use magazine pictures to help others understand the meaning of your poster, or you may draw your own pictures. All art supplies are on the table in the back of the room. If you need my help, ask me. When you are finished, we will hang the posters in the cafeteria.

After all the students have completed their posters, each student is given a turn displaying his to the class and discussing the slogan portrayed in his poster.

Note: Those students who do not live with their immediate families may tell of responsibilities that they have to others in their homes. They may make posters depicting the responsibilities discussed.

MATERIALS: Paper houses cut into pieces; paper; bulletin board; thumbtacks

PROCEDURE 1:

The students are seated in a semicircle, facing the bulletin board.   The teacher begins:

A few days ago, we talked about the word "responsibility." Can anyone tell us what the word means?

The teacher pauses to allow the students to define the word in their own terms.

After the word "responsibility" has been defined, the teacher explains:

We have talked about the word "responsibility" and about the ways we can be responsible people in our own homes. Soon each of you will have a home of your own. Some of you will have children. I want each of you to think of ways that you can be a responsible parent. I will give each of you a piece of paper and parts of a house. As you tell us one way in which you can be a responsible parent, you will begin to build a house. Let's let Joey begin.

Joey, what is one way you can be a responsible parent?

Joey responds:

I can see that my children get the right things to eat.

The teacher replies:

Yes, Joey, parents are responsible for seeing that their children eat the right foods. Here is a part of your house. Paste this in the center of your paper.

This activity continues until each student has had the opportunity to state responsibilities necessary in forming his own family unit and to complete the building of his house.

Each student may display his house on the bulletin board after its completion.

MATERIALS: Chalk; chalkboard; eraser

PROCEDURE 2:

The students are seated in a semicircle, facing the chalkboard. The teacher begins:

We have been talking about the word "responsibility." Soon you may be responsible for the
health, happiness, safety, shelter, income
and education of your own families. I have
written the words "health," "happiness,"
"safety," "shelter," "income" and "education"
on the board. We will define or tell what
the words mean. We will talk about each of
these words.

The teacher guides the students in defining the words on the
board. After the words have been defined and discussed, the
teacher explains:

Now that you understand what the words on the
board mean, we will talk about how we can be
responsible for each of these areas in our
own families. I want each of you to tell one
way in which you can be responsible for the
health of your own family. I will write the
responsibilities on the board under the word
"health." Who can tell one way in which we
can be responsible for the health of our own
families?

The teacher lists the responsibilities identified by the
students under the word "health." After each student has
had several opportunities to contribute, the teacher moves
on to the next area of responsibility, happiness. The
teacher and students discuss the various responsibilities
for happiness, and the teacher writes the responses on the
chalkboard.

This activity continues until each student can identify
responsibilities necessary for the six areas listed on the
board.

SECTION 3

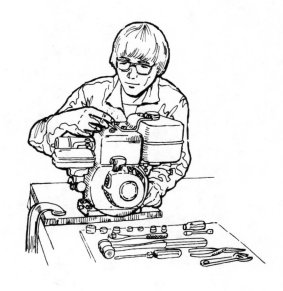

I Am a Worker

WORK-RELATED VOCABULARY

application form
appointment
bonus
check
coffee break
deduction
dependents
dues
employee
employer
employment agency
experience
factory
fired
fringe benefits
full-time
health insurance
interview
labor
labor unions
lay off
life insurance
minimum wage
pay

part-time
pay check
products
profit sharing
punch in-out
raise
references
resign
retirement
safety rules
seniority
skills
social security
strike
taxes
time clock
time off
vocational counselor
W-2 forms
wage
will train
withholding
workmen's compensation
work schedule

OBJECTIVE: Each Student Can Demonstrate an Understanding of the Concept, "Work"

MATERIALS: Paper; felt-tipped pen; large job jar; chalk; chalkboard; eraser

PROCEDURE 1:

The students are seated in a semicircle, facing the chalkboard. The teacher begins:

Today we are going to define the word "work."
Remember, when we define a word, we tell what
it means. I will write the word "work" on
the board. I will draw a line under the word
"work." Who can define the word?

Jill, please tell us what the word "work"
means.

Jill responds:

It is a job.

The teacher writes the word "job" under the word "work" and
then comments:

Yes, Jill, work is a job that we do.

Who else can describe work? Let me help you.
Suppose I want to move all the furniture in

this room to Mr. Piligrin's room next door. Would that be an easy or a hard job?

How would you describe that job, Ann?

Ann responds:

It would be hard to do.

The teacher replies:

Yes, Ann, sometimes work is hard to do. It requires much effort. I will write the word "effort" under the word "job." Fred, how would you describe the word "work"?

Fred answers:

It is something we have to do.

The teacher remarks:

Yes, Fred, some work we have to do. Sometimes we must work to earn money. Sometimes we must work very hard at school so we can learn to earn money. Sometimes we must work very hard in our homes to help each member of our families and ourselves.

Let's think of different types of work we do in our own homes. As you name the different types of work, I will write them on pieces of paper. I will then put the papers in our job jar.

As the students respond by telling different kinds of work they do at home, the teacher records these on paper slips and places the slips in the job jar. When the students cannot think of any more kinds of work they do at home, the teacher comments:

Now we will think of the ways we work at
school. As you tell the different types of
work we do at school, I will write the types
of work on the slips and put the slips of
paper in the job jar.

As the students tell the different types of work they do at
school, the teacher records these on the slips of paper and
places the slips in the job jar. When the students have told
of many different types of work, the teacher continues:

Sometimes we say that we have a job after
school or that we work after school. Many
times we are paid for what we do. Let's
think of all the types of work we could do
after school. As you think of these types
of work, I will write them down and put them
in our job jar.

After the students have indicated many types of afterschool
jobs, the teacher holds up the jar and says:

Look at all the types of work we do. If we
did all these jobs, we would accomplish many
things. I want each of you to think of
another type of work. Tomorrow you will tell
what type of work you thought of, and I will
write it on this paper for our job jar. Let's
see if we can fill the job jar tomorrow.

This activity continues the next day, with each student
having the opportunity to contribute another type of work,
thus demonstrating an understanding of the concept, "work."

MATERIALS: Chalk; chalkboard; eraser

PROCEDURE 2:

The students are seated at their desks, facing the chalkboard.
The teacher writes the word "work" on the board and explains:

> We use the word "work" every day in many
> different ways. I might say: "Ann is working
> so hard," or "I'll get to work on that" or "I
> can't go, I have too much work to do." We
> can work in different ways. Sometimes we work
> very hard with our bodies. When we work with
> our bodies, we use "physical" effort. Some-
> times we work very hard with our brains, then
> we use "mental" effort. The thing we are
> trying to do or to accomplish we call our
> goal. I will write a definition of "work" on
> the chalkboard.

The teacher writes the following information on the chalkboard: "Work is mental and/or physical effort to reach a
goal." After he has written the definition of work on the
board, he again explains the terms "physical" and "mental."
Then he says:

> Watch as I put on the board words that will
> help us to understand better the word "work."

The teacher then writes and again explains:

> Work = Task + Mental and/or Physical Effort
> + Goal.

The teacher continues:

> Look at this jar. It is filled with jobs
> that we have all done. The types of jobs
> are written on pieces of paper. I will pick
> one from the jar. I have picked "washing
> dishes." So under "Task," I will write
> "washing dishes."

Now who can tell what physical effort I use
to wash dishes? Ann? Yes, Ann, I must clear
the dishes of the food remaining on them,
stack them, fill a sink with soap and water,
wash and rinse each dish. Excellent.

Tom, what mental effort do I use to wash
dishes? Very good, Tom. I must be careful
to stack them so they don't break, I must
look to see if they are clean and rinsed.

What is my goal, Tom, in washing dishes?
Yes, I want clean, dry, unchipped dishes.
There is much work involved in washing
dishes.

Fred, you may pick a slip of paper from the
job jar. You have picked "paint the kitchen."
So under "Task," I will write "paint the
kitchen." What physical effort must you make
to paint the kitchen, Fred?

Fred's answer should include "buy paint and brush"; "wash
down walls"; "clean brushes"; "remove furniture and dishes."

Under mental effort, Fred's answer should include "select
color"; "buy the best paint at the lowest possible price";
"be careful not to drip it on the floor"; "open a window
while you are painting"; "keep small children away from
paint."

Under goal, Fred's answer should indicate a clean, attractive
room.

This activity continues until each student has had the
opportunity to demonstrate an understanding of the concept,
"work."

OBJECTIVE: Each Student Can Identify Occupations Depicted in Pictures

MATERIALS: Large picture showing grocery store employees at work; bulletin board; thumbtacks

PROCEDURE 1:

The students are seated in a semicircle, facing the bulletin board. A large picture of a grocery store is posted on the bulletin board. The teacher points to the picture on the bulletin board and says:

> This is a picture of a grocery store and of the people who work there. Raise your hand if you have been to a grocery store.

After the students have raised their hands, the teacher continues:

> Several of you have been shopping in a grocery store. Who would like to tell about this trip to the grocery?

After the students have had an opportunity to discuss their experiences in the grocery store, the teacher comments:

> You have told many interesting stories about your experiences at the grocery store. Now let's look at the picture of the grocery store on the bulletin board. We see many people at work in the grocery. I will name and point to the workers in the picture. I

will tell about each person's job. You may
wish to tell more about the workers in the
picture. After we have finished talking
about each of the workers, I want you to
point to the workers and name the jobs that
they do.

The teacher identifies and points to the workers in the
picture. Next, the teacher gives a job description of each
of the workers in the picture. A discussion follows in
which the students are encouraged to relate personal experiences and to contribute additional information or observations concerning job descriptions of the workers in the
picture.

This activity continues until each student has had the
opportunity to identify the workers and to describe the type
of work they do.

Note: The teacher may wish to use the same procedure in
identifying other occupations within the experience
realm of the students. These would include occupations relating to restaurants, banks, dry cleaning
establishments, department stores. The teacher should
introduce new vocabulary related to these occupations,
discuss the words with the students and have the
students use the words.

If large activity pictures of workers in various occupations are not available from commercial language
or reading kits, the teacher may have to use several
small pictures depicting workers in each occupation.

MATERIALS: Visitors who will discuss occupations with students;
            pictures depicting each occupation discussed; bulletin
            board; thumbtacks

PROCEDURE 2:

(Prior to this lesson, the teacher has arranged for the vocational rehabilitation counselor, the guidance counselor and/or
people from the community who hire students to visit and to
discuss employment available and appropriate to the students'
potential skill and ability levels. The teacher has also
borrowed or collected pictures depicting the occupations to
be discussed and has placed them on the bulletin board.)

After the visitors have discussed employment opportunities
with the students, the teacher comments:

    We have talked about many jobs that may in-
    terest you. On the bulletin board are dis-
    played pictures showing workers doing the
    jobs we have discussed. I want each of you
    to identify all the jobs shown in the pic-
    tures. After you have identified all the
    jobs, you may tell us which job you are
    interested in and why you are interested in
    it.

This activity continues until each student can identify the
occupations depicted in the pictures and has had the opportunity to tell about the occupation he is interested in.

MATERIALS: Area of classroom designed as workers' store with
items the students may purchase; price tags marked
in dollar units, one on each item; play one dollar
bills; working vocabulary list; chalk; chalkboard;
eraser

PROCEDURE 1:

The students are seated in a semicircle, facing the chalkboard. The teacher begins:

We have been talking about work. We have
talked about the meaning of the word "work"
and about different types of work we have
done. Today we will talk about words that
the worker will need to know. You will learn
many new words. For every word that you
learn, you will earn one play dollar. When
we have finished our lesson today, you may
take your money to the workers' store. You
may use your dollars to buy something from
the store. Watch as I write the first word
on the board.

The teacher writes the word "employee" on the board and
explains:

I have written the word "employee" on the
board. An "employee" is a person who works

111

for another person or for a company. An
employee is a worker.

Now I will write another word on the board.
The word is "employer." An "employer" is the
person or company for which the "employee"
works.

Marie, your father is a worker. He is an
employee of a company. What is that company?

Marie responds:

It is the telephone company.

The teacher comments:

Very good, Marie. Your father works for the
telephone company. He is an employee of the
telephone company. The telephone company is
his employer. Remember--an employer is a
person or a company for whom the employee
works.

Now, Marie, let me tell you about Raymond.
He works in Mr. Jones' restaurant. Who is
the employee?

Marie answers:

Raymond is.

The teacher remarks:

That's fine. Who is Raymond's employer?

Marie responds:

Mr. Jones is.

The teacher observes:

> Well done, Marie. Now let's talk about
> another new word.

After the teacher has introduced 10 words, written them on
the board, defined them and discussed them with the students,
he summarizes by saying:

> We have talked about all the words on the
> board. I will point to them and read them
> to you.

After the teacher has read the words to the class, he
continues:

> Jill, tell us the word that means "a person
> who works for another person or for a
> company."

Jill replies:

> It is "employee."

The teacher comments:

> Good, Jill. Now come to the board and point
> to the word "employee."

This activity continues until each student has had an opportunity to supply the appropriate vocabulary word when
given the definition of the term. For each correct response,
the teacher gives the student a play dollar which may be
used to purchase the item of his choice from the workers'
store at the end of this activity.

Note: It will be necessary to carry out this activity over
       a number of days. The teacher may decide to use all
       or some of the vocabulary words provided on page 100,
       and/or he may supply his own terms and definitions.

MATERIALS: Area of classroom designed as workers' store with
items the students may purchase; price tags marked
in dollar units, one on each item; play one dollar
bills; working vocabulary, printed on 3" x 5" cards,
one word per card; shoe box; chalk; chalkboard;
eraser

PROCEDURE 2:

(Prior to this activity, the teacher has printed the words
to be discussed on 3" x 5" cards and has placed the cards
in a shoe box.)

The students are seated at their desks, facing the chalkboard. The teacher begins:

Today we are going to talk about words which
workers should know. We are going to define
these words. Remember, to define is to tell
what the words mean. Watch as I write the
first word on the board.

The teacher writes the word "employee" on the chalkboard
and explains:

I have written the word "employee" on the
board. An employee is a worker. An employee
is a person who works for another person or
for a company. For example, I am an employee.
I work for the school system.

The teacher continues to write vocabulary words on the board,
to define the words and to discuss the words with the students until there are twice as many words on the board as
there are students in the class.

After the teacher has discussed all the words with the students, he picks up the shoe box and explains:

Each of the words we have discussed is written
on a card which is in this shoe box. When I
call your name, pick two cards from the box.
If you cannot read the words on your cards, I

114

will read them for you. When you have your
cards and know what the words are, take the
cards back to your desk and be seated.

After each student has picked two cards and placed them on
his desk, the teacher says:

Raise your hand if you have the word
"employee" written on one of your cards.

After the student who has the word "employee" has raised her
hand, the teacher comments:

Jane has the word "employee." Jane, can
you tell us what the word means? What does
the word "employee" mean?

Jane answers:

An employee is a worker.

The teacher replies:

Very good. An employee is a worker. Whom
might the employee work for?

Jane responds:

He probably works for a person or for a
company.

The teacher comments:

Well done. You can define the word. Now
tell the class what word is printed on the
other card.

Jane responds:

It is "wages."

The teacher asks:

What does the word "wages" mean?

Jane answers:

Wages are pay you get for working.

The teacher remarks:

Yes, Jane. Wages are pay you receive for
working. You get paid a certain amount of
money for each hour you work. This money
is called your wage.

Jane has defined her two words. Jane, please
return the words to the box and then be
seated. Here is two dollars, your wage for
your work.

After each student has had an opportunity to define his
words and to return the words to the shoe box, each student
selects two more words from the box.

This activity continues until each student can define all
the vocabulary introduced. After the lesson has been completed, each student is allowed to purchase items from the
store with the money he has earned.

Note: Several class sessions will be necessary to complete
this activity. The teacher may add vocabulary to the
list provided on page 100, and/or he may delete those
terms that are inappropriate.

OBJECTIVE: Each Student Can Identify Tasks Related to Different Occupations

MATERIALS: 10 pictures of workers engaged in various job-related activities; numbers 1 through 10 made of construction paper; number cards with the numbers 1 through 10, one number per card; bulletin board; thumbtacks

PROCEDURE 1:

(Prior to this activity, the students, assisted by the teacher, have made the numbers 1 through 10 out of construction paper. The teacher has printed the same numbers on the cards.)

The students are seated in a semicircle, facing the bulletin board. The teacher begins:

Today we are going to talk about 10 different jobs. We will talk about what tasks workers must perform for each of the jobs we discuss. I will put pictures of people doing the jobs we will talk about on the bulletin board. Watch as I put up the first picture.

After the teacher has tacked the first picture on the board, he aids the students in identifying the occupation portrayed in the picture and in identifying the tasks required for the job.

We have discussed the first job picture on the board. I will put the number 1 beside it.

117

The teacher places the number 1, made of construction paper, beside the first picture. He continues tacking the pictures on the board, helping the students identify the jobs and the tasks involved and placing the number beside each picture until all 10 job pictures have been identified and discussed. Then he remarks:

> We have talked about 10 jobs. I have placed pictures of people doing these jobs on the board, and I have placed a number beside each picture. Now I will give each of you a number.

The teacher gives each student a card which has one number written on it. The teacher says:

> Each of you has a number. Patti, please come to the board and match your number to one on the board.

If Patti is unable to match her number to the corresponding number on the board, the teacher says:

> Patti, the number written on your card is 5. I will point to the number 5 on the board. Watch as I hold the number on your card next to the number on the board. They are alike. They match. They are both 5's. Now I will return your card. You may find the number on the board that matches your number.

After Patti has matched her number to one on the board, the teacher remarks:

> Well done, Patti. You have matched your number. Now look at the picture beside your number. Tell us what job the person in the picture is doing. Be sure to use sentences when you tell us.

Patti responds:

He is working. He is a butcher.

The teacher replies:

> Very good, Patti. The picture shows a
> butcher at work. Please tell us what a
> butcher does.

Patti responds:

> A butcher cuts meat. He puts the meat in
> a package. He cleans up the mess.

The teacher comments:

> That is a very good description, Patti. You
> have told us what the butcher does. You may
> return to your seat.

This activity continues until each student can describe, in
simple sentences, tasks related to different occupations.

MATERIALS: Chalk; chalkboard; eraser

PROCEDURE 2:

    The students are seated at their desks, facing the chalk-
board. The teacher begins:

        I am going to list the titles of several jobs
        on the board.

    The teacher then writes the titles of several jobs on the
chalkboard and identifies the words for the students. The
teacher explains:

        Now that you know what the jobs are that I
        have listed on the board, I will tell about
        the duties associated with one of these
        jobs. When you know which job I am talking
        about, raise your hand.

    After the students have associated job responsibilities with
job titles, the teacher erases the board and explains:

        When people are looking for a job, they often
        look in the want ads of the newspaper under
        employment. The job title, a job description
        and the name of the person to call about the
        job are often found in the newspaper want ads.
        Today we are going to write want ads for the
        jobs we have discussed.

        Leonard, you may begin the activity. What
        job would you like to tell about?

    After Leonard has selected a job title, the teacher remarks:

        Leonard will help me write a want ad for a
        job as a salad maker in a restaurant or a
        cafeteria. I will write the words "salad
        maker" on the board.

Leonard, you may tell us the responsibilities
of a salad maker. Remember to use sentences
to tell about the responsibilities for this
job. I will write the responsibilities for
the job on the board.

Leonard responds:

A salad maker washes the vegetables. A salad
maker peels the vegetables. A salad maker
cuts the vegetables. A salad maker mixes the
salad together.

The teacher observes:

You have named many duties of a salad maker,
but not all the duties. Rita, what are some
other responsibilities of a salad maker?

Rita answers:

A salad maker must read and follow a recipe.
A salad maker must clean up his mess.

The teacher comments:

Yes, Rita, you have told us other duties of a
salad maker. I will write the duties you and
Leonard have named on the chalkboard under
"salad maker."

After the teacher has listed the duties required for the job
of salad maker on the board, he reads them to the students
and remarks:

We know what a salad maker does. Where do
you think we might go to look for a job as
a salad maker? We will need that information
for our want ad.

William, what are some places that might hire
a salad maker?

After William has named a number of local establishments
that might hire salad makers, the teacher selects the name
of one establishment to be included in the want ad. The
teacher observes:

Now our want ad tells us the title of the job
that is available, the duties of the job and
the place where the job is available. Let's
choose another job to write about.

This activity continues until each student is able to
describe, in simple sentences, tasks related to the occupations being discussed.

OBJECTIVE: Each Student Can Describe a Work Experience

MATERIALS: Six 12" x 8" cards, with the words, "what," "when," "where," "how," "who," "why," written, one word on each card; job jar

PROCEDURE 1:

(Prior to this activity, the teacher has written different job titles on slips of paper, one per slip, and has placed them in the job jar.)

The students are seated in a semicircle. The teacher begins:

> For several days, we have been discussing the word "work." Today each of us will describe work we have done. If you have trouble remembering a job you have done, you may go to the job jar and take a job slip. If you need help reading what is written on the paper, let me know.

After each of the students has decided on a particular job, the teacher explains:

> Look at the cards that I am holding. This first one has the word "what" written on it. When I show you this card, you will tell us <u>what</u> job you did. Remember to use sentences when you answer.

> The second card has the word "when" written on it. When I hold up this card, you will tell us <u>when</u> you did the work.

The third card has the word "where." When I hold up this card, you will tell us <u>where</u> you worked.

The fourth card has the word "how." When I hold it up, you will tell us <u>how</u> you worked.

The fifth card has the word "who." When you see this card, you will tell us <u>who</u> was working with you--if you were not working alone.

The sixth card has the word "why." When you see this card, you will tell us <u>why</u> you did your job.

John, you may begin.

The teacher holds up the card with "what" and asks:

What work did you do, John?

John answers:

I washed the car.

The teacher holds up the card with "when" and asks:

When did you wash the car?

John answers:

Last Saturday.

The teacher corrects him by saying:

Remember to use a sentence, John. Say, "I washed the car last Saturday."

John repeats the patterned sentence.

The teacher holds up the card with "where" and asks:

Where did you wash the car?

John answers:

I washed it in the driveway.

The teacher holds up the card with "how" and asks:

How did you wash the car?

John answers:

I put soap and water on it. I scrubbed it
with rags. I rinsed it with the hose.

The teacher remarks:

Good, John. Now look at this card. It has
the word "why." Why did you wash the car?

John responds:

My mother asked me to wash it.

The teacher commends him by saying:

You have answered all the questions. You
have described the work you did. Well done,
John.

The teacher chooses another student to answer the six
question cards. This activity continues until each student
can relate a work experience, by answering "what," "when,"
"where," "how," "who," "why."

MATERIALS: Seven 12" x 8" cards, with the words, "what," "when,"
              "where," "how," "who," "why," "feelings," written,
              one word on each card; job jar; bulletin board;
              thumbtacks

PROCEDURE 2:

   (Prior to this activity, the teacher has written different
   jobs on slips of paper, one job per slip, and has placed
   them in the job jar.)

   The students are seated in a semicircle, facing the bulletin
   board. The teacher tacks the cards to the bulletin board
   and reads the words on the cards to the students. The
   teacher explains:

      Today we are going to tell about jobs we have
      done. Let's see how many of you will be able
      to tell all about your jobs. You must include
      what you did; when you did it; where you did
      it; how you did it; who helped you, if anyone;
      why you did it; how you felt about it. You
      may look at the cards on the board to remind
      you to include all the important facts.

      John, you may begin. Pick a slip from the job
      jar. If you have never done the job, return
      the slip to the job jar and pick another.

   John picks a slip from the jar and thinks for a few moments.
   Then he says:

      I shoveled snow with Ted last night. We used
      our new snow shovels. We shoveled all the
      walks and the driveway at Mr. Barrett's house.
      Mrs. Barrett gave us hot cocoa when we were
      finished. We were cold and tired, but we felt
      good because the walks and driveway looked
      good.

   The teacher remarks:

126

Excellent, John. Did he forget anything, Mary?

Mary answers:

He forgot to say who helped him.

The teacher replies:

Did you forget that, John?

John answers:

No, I said I worked with Ted.

The teacher replies:

Yes, you did. We will listen more carefully.

This activity continues until each student has had the opportunity to tell about a job he has done, by including "what," "when," "where," "how," "who," "why," "how he felt."

Note: Jobs the students may tell about may include, but need not be limited to, washing clothes, filling gas tanks, baiting hooks for fishermen, painting houses, parking cars, packing meat, milking cows, studying lessons, making beds, raking leaves, collecting letters, feeding animals, washing windows, bathing pets, pushing wheelchairs, planting seeds, mowing lawns, using tools, arranging flowers.

OBJECTIVE: Each Student Can Verbalize Skills Necessary for a Specific Job Available to Him

---

MATERIALS: Pictures of workers engaged in types of jobs available to the students; bulletin board; thumbtacks

PROCEDURE 1:

(Prior to this activity, the teacher has collected pictures of workers engaged in jobs available to the students and has placed one picture on the bulletin board.)

The students are seated in a semicircle, facing the bulletin board. The teacher begins:

Today we are going to look at pictures of workers. The workers are doing jobs that you may do some day. Look at the picture on the board. Who can tell about the worker in the picture?

Jan, what can you tell us about the worker in the picture?

Jan responds:

It is a girl. She is making hair curlers.

The teacher comments:

Yes, Jan, she is making hair curlers. She
works at a workshop. Her name is Rita. Rita
works very hard. She works with her hands.
She must be able to put together the small
pieces of the curlers. She must be able to
use her hands quickly and carefully.

She must have good vision. She must be able
to see the small pieces with which she works.

We can see that Rita needs to be able to
work quickly. She must make many curlers
each hour.

We can see that Rita needs to be able to
work with her hands. She must be able to
move small parts of the curlers.

Rita must have good eyes. She must be able
to see the small parts of the curlers.

Rita needs many skills for her job. A <u>skill</u>
is an <u>ability</u>, being able to do something
special. Rita has many skills. She has good
vision to see the small parts of the curlers.
She is able to work quickly and carefully
with her hands.

Now let's look at another picture of a worker.
Try to tell what skills this worker may need
for his job.

The teacher removes Rita's picture and places another picture
of a worker engaged in a job-related activity on the bulletin
board. The teacher instructs the students to determine the
skills necessary for the specific job represented in the
picture.

This activity continues until each student has had the opportunity to verbalize the skills necessary for a specific
job available to him.

<u>MATERIALS</u>:   Paper; pencils; chalk; chalkboard; eraser

<u>PROCEDURE</u> <u>2</u>:

The students are seated at their desks, facing the chalkboard.
The teacher explains:

> Today we are going to talk about skills that
> you might need for different jobs. A <u>skill</u>
> is a special <u>ability</u>. I am going to separate
> you into three groups. The first group will
> tell what the jobs are that you might be able
> to work at in a restaurant. For each type of
> work named, the group should list the special
> skills needed for each job.
>
> The next group will tell us what jobs might
> be available in a motel. They will tell
> about the special skills needed for each job.
>
> The last group will tell us what jobs might
> be available in a gas station. They will
> tell about the special skills needed for each
> job.
>
> Now I will assign you to groups. You will
> have 15 minutes to list the jobs available
> and the skills needed for each job. I will
> visit each group to offer ideas and help if
> it is needed.

After the three groups have compiled lists of available
jobs and skills related to them, each group shares its
ideas with the class. The teacher encourages all the members of each group to contribute to the discussion.

After the three groups have presented their lists, the
teacher summarizes the findings of each group. The teacher
says:

> We have talked about many different jobs
> available to you. I will write the names
> of the jobs we have talked about on the
> board.

After the teacher has written the words on the board and has read them to the class, the teacher continues:

>Now I will point to one of the jobs on the board and name it. Raise your hand when you can tell the skills necessary for that job.

This activity continues until each student can verbalize the skills necessary for specific jobs available to him.

OBJECTIVE: Each Student Can Demonstrate an Understanding of the Procedures Necessary for Finding a Job

---

MATERIALS: Card table; toy phone; newspaper employment want ads, one ad for each student; pad of paper; pencil; overhead projector and stand

PROCEDURE 1:

(Prior to this activity, the teacher has placed a card table and a toy phone at the front of the room to one side. On the other side he has placed the overhead projector on a stand.)

The students are seated at their desks, facing the overhead projector. The teacher has newspaper employment want ads, one ad for each member of the class. The teacher begins:

Today we are going to talk about jobs that are listed in the want ads of the newspaper. I will put an ad on the projector and will read it to you. Listen carefully.

Look at the top of the column. Written here are the words "Help Wanted." This is the part of the want ad that tells us what job is available.

Now look under this column heading. This is the want ad. The want ad says:

            Buzzy's Restaurant
            Openings for: Dishwasher,
            waitress--AM shift, busboys.
            Please call 845-9090. Seminole.

      From the ad we know the name of the employer.
      We know the jobs that are available. We know
      the phone number to call to make an appoint-
      ment to see the employer.

      John, you may come to the table. You may
      apply for this job. What is the name of the
      restaurant that you are going to call?

John responds:

      It is Buzzy's Restaurant.

The teacher replies:

      Very good, John, What is the job that
      interests you?

John answers:

      It is dishwasher.

The teacher asks:

      What is the phone number of the restaurant?
      Please read it for the class.

John responds:

      It is 845-9090.

The teacher then asks:

John, what will you say when you call the
restaurant?

John replies:

I'll tell them I want to be a dishwasher.

The teacher comments:

Yes, John, but first, you should tell them
you are calling about the job in the newspaper.
You should then tell them that you want to be
a dishwasher. You should ask when you can
make an appointment to talk to them at the
restaurant. You will need to ask them the
location of the restaurant, the address, if
you are to go there. Use the pad of paper
and the pencil to record these. You may now
dial the number, and we will practice.

The teacher guides John through the procedure for obtaining
a job. When they have completed the procedure, the teacher
gives each student his own want ad and guides each one through
the job process procedure.

This activity continues until each student can demonstrate an
understanding of the procedures that are necessary for finding
employment.

Note: The teacher should also introduce and explain to the
       students want ads that request that the applicant
       apply in person. The teacher may also wish to arrange
       for a vocational rehabilitation counselor and a state
       employment agency agent to speak to the students con-
       cerning alternative ways of seeking employment.

MATERIALS: Guest lecturers, one lecturer from the vocational rehabilitation agency, one from the state employment agency and one from a newspaper; arrangements for field trip (optional)

PROCEDURE 2:

(Prior to this activity, the teacher has arranged for a guest lecturer from each of the following: vocational rehabilitation agency, state employment agency and newspaper, and, if possible, has arranged a field trip to each of these places. The teacher asks each speaker to talk on "Helping You to Find a Job," utilizing the following suggestions:

1. Newspaper Representative:

   a. Where to find the want ads for employment.

   b. How to read abbreviations in the ads.

   c. How to place a want ad offering your specific skills.

   d. How to respond to ads.

   e. What information the employer will need from the students.

2. Vocational Rehabilitation Counselor:

   a. Specific businesses in which the agency places students.

   b. Types of jobs offered to students.

   c. Skills necessary for specific jobs.

   d. Duties related to specific jobs.

   e. Procedures for securing employment.

   f. Ways the counselor works with students to secure employment and to succeed on the job.

3. State Employment Agency Agent:

   a. The function of the agency.

   b. Ways the agency aids the student.

   c. Procedures the student should follow in applying for employment through the agency.

   d. Special aid the agency offers, such as unemployment compensation, counseling, etc.

   e. Information the agency will need about the students in order to help them in securing employment.

Each speaker should be given an entire class session in which to present ways in which he or his agency might assist the students in finding employment. After each session, there should be a question and answer period.

To reinforce information presented by the three speakers, the teacher may take the students to the agencies and to the newspaper to observe, and perhaps take part in, procedures for finding employment.

The teacher may wish to use the information gained from the talks and the field trips to determine the students' degree of understanding of the procedures involved in finding a job.

OBJECTIVE: Each Student Can Role Play a Job Interview

MATERIALS: Wallet-sized cards, one for each student, with the
              words, "name," "address," "phone," "social security
              number," "birth date," printed on each card; chalk;
              chalkboard; eraser

PROCEDURE 1:

The students are seated at their desks, facing the chalkboard. The teacher distributes a card to each student and
says:

    Today we are going to prepare for a job inter-
    view. I will write the word "interview" on
    the chalkboard.

After the teacher has written the word on the board, he
continues:

    An interview is a meeting to find out informa-
    tion. The employer or boss wants to find out
    if you will be a good worker. You want to
    find out if you will like the job, or if you
    can do the job. Each of you must be sure you
    will be able to answer questions about your-
    self. Look at the cards I gave you. Please
    fill in all the information about yourself.
    If you need help, raise your hand.

When all the cards have been completed, the teacher tells
the students that they may refer to them during the activity.
The teacher explains:

Let us suppose that the sheltered workshop
at the phone company has asked Rosemary to
come for an interview. I will act out the
part of Mr. Taylor, who runs the workshop
and who will be asking the questions.

Rosemary, you may bring your card and come
here.

At the beginning of the "interview," the teacher explains
the duties, skills, responsibilities and benefits associated
with the job. The teacher continues:

Rosemary, I think that you would be a good
worker. Do you have any questions about
the job?

The teacher encourages Rosemary to ask specific questions
regarding employment. If Rosemary is unable to direct
specific questions to the teacher spontaneously, members of
the class should be encouraged to help her in formulating
questions.

After general information concerning the job has been obtained through this question-answer technique, the teacher
comments:

I have decided to hire you. I will need to
know many things about you. I will need to
write information on your record. I will
need to know your full name, your address,
your phone number, your social security
number and your birth date. Will you please
give me this information?

The teacher then tells Rosemary that she may refer to the
card given to her earlier to supply the information. The
teacher asks:

Rosemary, what is your full name?

The teacher instructs Rosemary to supply all the information
asked for and encourages her to use simple patterned sentences in giving her answers.

This activity continues until each student has had the opportunity to role play a job interview.

Note: Some students may not have a social security number. The teacher should instruct them as to how to obtain one.

MATERIALS: Chalk; chalkboard; eraser

PROCEDURE 2:

(Prior to this activity, each student has completed a sample job application form. The teacher has evaluated and returned the form to each student. The form should include name, address, phone, date of birth, social security number, schooling, experience, references.)

The students are seated in a semicircle, facing the chalkboard. The teacher explains:

You are ready for a very important lesson in your study of jobs. You are going to role play job interviews. You have all completed application forms. You have applied for jobs by letter. Today you will apply for jobs in person. You do this in an interview. An interview is always important. It is important to the employer, the person who is looking for help. The employer will want to know many things about you. He will ask many questions. Think of all the questions an employer could ask you during a job interview.

As the students respond, the teacher writes their questions on the chalkboard. The questions may include:

1. Why do you want to work here?
2. What experience have you had?
3. Why did you leave your last job?
4. When could you begin work?
5. What salary do you expect?
6. Do you have references?
7. How old are you?
8. Why did you leave school?
9. Have you ever been arrested?

When each student has contributed a question and has also demonstrated the ability to answer one, the teacher erases the questions from the board and says:

Now, which questions should you ask the
employer? When you think of a question, I
will write it on the board.

The students' responses should include:

1. What are the hours?
2. What is the salary?
3. What are the fringe benefits?
4. Do you pay weekly? Monthly?
5. What are the job requirements?

The teacher follows the same format used with the employer's
questions. When all the questions have been compiled and
responses formed, the teacher explains:

You will now role play an interview. Remember, every person who interviews you will
be different. There is no set form or pattern. Suppose I am the owner of the Country
Inn, and I am looking for a busboy. John has
applied by letter, and I have sent for him
for an interview.

John, you may come to the front of the room
and help me to role play this interview.

After the teacher has enacted the interview with John, the
students evaluate the performance in terms of whether or not
John will get the job.

This activity continues until each student has had the opportunity to role play a job interview.

Note: As the students become comfortable in the role of
       employee, they may try the role of employer. This
       will reinforce the necessity of good communication
       on the part of the job seeker. Video tape, if
       available, is excellent for this evaluation process.
       As the students advance in interview communication
       skills, the teacher could ask potential employers to
       volunteer to role play with class members, for
       example, state employment interviewers; local store,
       restaurant, garage, newspaper people.

MATERIALS: Large cutout face of a boy named Ted; "happy faces,"
one for each student; work-related problem, with
three possible solutions, one of which is correct,
for each student; bulletin board; thumbtacks

PROCEDURE 1:

The students are seated in a semicircle, facing the bulletin
board. The teacher places a cutout face on the bulletin
board and explains:

Today we are going to talk about problems that
may happen at work. Look at the bulletin
board. On the board we see a picture of Ted.
Ted is a worker. Ted has a problem. I will
tell about Ted's problem. When I am finished
telling about Ted's problem, you may choose
the best way to solve Ted's problem. If you
choose the best answer to Ted's problem, you
will earn a "happy face" for helping Ted solve
his problem. Here is Ted's problem. Listen
carefully.

Ted works at the workshop. He puts together
hair curlers in the workshop. He tries very
hard to make as many hair curlers as he can.
Ted's problem is that one of the boys he
works with talks to him too much. This
makes Ted work too slowly.

The teacher continues:

Now we know Ted's problem. Listen as I give
you some possible solutions to Ted's problem.
After you have listened to each of the three
solutions, I will ask someone to choose the
best one. If you choose the best solution,
you will earn a "happy face." Listen
carefully.

Here is the first solution: Ted should look
for a new job.

Here is the second solution: Ted should ask
his boss to fire the boy.

Here is the third solution: Ted should tell
the boy that he will talk to him on his
coffee break and explain that when he talks
while he works he becomes confused and works
too slowly.

Ann Marie, please tell us which of the three
solutions is the best one.

Ann Marie says:

I think he should talk on his coffee break.
He can work faster when he is not talking.

The teacher remarks:

Very good. You have chosen the best solution.
You have earned a "happy face" for helping
Ted solve his problem.

The teacher should then discuss the alternative solutions
with the students. He should help them determine why the
alternative solutions were not the best one to the problem.

The teacher should give each student a work-related problem,
with three possible solutions. If the student gives the
best solution, the class members should discuss why the
solution he chose is better than the two alternative ones.
If the student does not choose the best solution, the class
members, aided by the teacher, should help him understand
why one of the other two would be a better solution to the
problem.

This activity continues until each student has had the opportunity to participate in solving a work-related problem, thus earning a "happy face."

MATERIALS: Job-related problems; chalk; chalkboard; eraser

PROCEDURE 2:

The students are seated at their desks, facing the chalk-board. The teacher explains:

> Today we are going to talk about problems
> which might happen on the job. Listen care-
> fully to each problem. I will ask several
> of you to tell us how you would solve the
> problem. I will write your solution on the
> board. I will ask one of you to decide
> which solution is the best and to tell why.
> Here is the first problem.

> Marie has just begun a new job. She works
> at a car wash. She dries the cars. As she
> works, she notices that one of the customers
> has left a package in the waiting area. What
> should Marie do?

The teacher writes the students' solutions to the problem on the bulletin board. After he has written a number of solu-tions on the board, he remarks:

> There are many possible solutions to Marie's
> problem. Let us pick the three best alter-
> natives from this list.

The teacher aids the students in their selection of the three most likely solutions. Then he remarks:

> We now have the three most likely solutions
> to Marie's problem. Listen as I read them
> to you. Choose the one you believe is the
> best. When I call on you, you may tell us
> why you think it is the best answer. Here
> are the solutions:

1. Marie should keep the package.

2. Marie should tell her friends that she found the package.

3. Marie should tell her boss that she found the package.

Joe, which do you think is the best answer?

Joe responds:

I would tell my boss that I found the package.

The teacher asks:

Why do you think that is the best thing to do?

Joe answers:

Marie can't keep the package. It belongs to someone else. Marie's boss will know what to do with the package. Marie's friends are too busy to help.

The teacher replies:

You have chosen the best answer. Now we will talk about another problem.

This activity continues until each student has had the opportunity to participate in a problem-solving activity related to work.

OBJECTIVE: Each Student Can Demonstrate an Understanding of the Concept, "Responsibility," in Regard to Work

---

MATERIALS: Overhead projector; pencil; ditto masters; duplicating paper; duplicator; stapler

PROCEDURE 1:

The students are seated at their desks, facing the overhead projector. The teacher places a blank ditto master sheet on the tray of the overhead projector. The teacher explains:

Each of you knows what it is to be a responsible person. Each of you knows ways to be a responsible family member. We are going to discuss ways that each of you might be a responsible worker.

We are going to make a booklet. The title of our booklet will be "We Are Responsible Workers." We will give copies of our booklet to members of the PTA at their next meeting. Now I will print the title on the paper on the projector.

After printing the title on the ditto master, the teacher removes the paper and replaces it with another. The teacher says:

I want each of you to think of ways to be a responsible worker.

Ann, tell us how you might demonstrate
responsibility while working.

Ann replied:

I would be on time.

The teacher responds:

Good, Ann. I will write "a responsible worker
is on time" on this paper.

As each student responds, the teacher writes the responses
on the ditto master.

Answers should include "A responsible worker is clean,"
". . . cheerful," ". . . hard-working," ". . . courteous,"
". . . loyal," ". . . thoughtful," ". . . ambitious,"
". . . well-groomed."

After each student has told how he might demonstrate responsible work behavior, the teacher asks for volunteers to
tell of specific incidents in which they have observed
responsible work behavior.

After each student has been able to demonstrate an understanding of the concept, "responsibility," in regard to
work, the teacher asks for volunteers to assist in the
duplication and construction of the booklets. Each student
should receive a copy of the booklet, and additional copies
should be put together for distribution to persons attending
the next PTA meeting.

MATERIALS: Local employers and former students, who are currently
             employed, to speak to the class; sheets of paper, one
             sheet for each group; pencils, one pencil for each
             group; materials to duplicate student articles for a
             class newspaper (these include ditto paper, duplica-
             tor, ditto masters, duplicator fluid, stapler);
             copies of class newspaper, one copy for each student

PROCEDURE 2:

   (Prior to this activity, the teacher has arranged for local
   employers to speak to the students on the topic of worker
   responsibility. The teacher has also arranged for former
   students, who are currently employed, to tell of specific
   examples of how they have demonstrated responsibility while
   working.)

   The teacher begins by saying:

        We have very important guests today. Some of
        our guests are employers. They will talk
        about workers' responsibilities. Some of our
        guests are employees. They will tell about
        ways in which they demonstrate responsibility
        at their various jobs. Listen very carefully
        to each of our speakers.

   After all the guests have spoken, the teacher thanks them.
   Then, to the students, he says:

        Now I will assign each of you to a group.
        Each group will be responsible for inter-
        viewing one of our guests. Each group
        should ask the guest how workers might show
        responsibility while working. The group
        may then choose one member to list ways a
        person may show he is a responsible worker.
        I will give each group a pencil and paper.
        Later, each group will use the information
        gathered to write an article which will be
        published in our newspaper.

   After the interviews have been completed, the teacher thanks
   the guests again, and the guests leave.

153

The teacher tells the students:

> It is time to write articles for the class
> newspaper. In each article, the word
> "responsibility" should be defined. In each
> article, ways to demonstrate responsibility
> as workers should be discussed.
>
> When all the articles have been completed,
> a member of each group may read a story to
> the class. After all the articles have been
> read, I will collect them and will reproduce
> them in the class newspaper. Each of you
> will receive a newspaper. Each of you may
> take it home for your family members to read.

After all the articles have been collected, the teacher
remarks:

> We have talked about ways that we, as workers,
> might demonstrate responsibility. Now I
> would like for each of you to name one way a
> person might show that he is a responsible
> worker.

This activity continues until each student can demonstrate
an understanding of the concept, "responsibility," in regard
to work.

SECTION 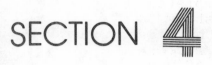 4

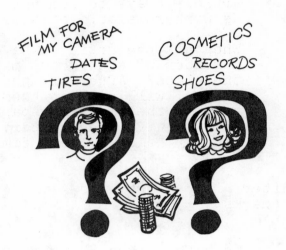

I Am a Consumer

CONSUMER-RELATED VOCABULARY

advertisement
appliance
bait and switch
bankruptcy
bargain
bill
buy
cash
cash-and-carry
charge
check
clearance
clerk
consumer
cost
coupon
credit
customer
discount
inventory

inventory clearance
layaway
limited quantity
90 days
price
purchase
refund
return
sales
salesman
sales slip
savings
special
trade
trade-in
two-for-one sale
value
warranty
white sale

```
┌────────────────────────────────────────────────────────────────┐
│  OBJECTIVE:  Each Student Can Demonstrate an Understanding of the Concept,  │
│              "Consumer"                                                       │
└────────────────────────────────────────────────────────────────┘
```

MATERIALS: Large pictures, one picture of each of the following:
               a house, food, clothing, furniture, an automobile, a
               doctor and a mechanic; magazines and pairs of scissors,
               one of each for each student; bulletin board; thumb-
               tacks

PROCEDURE 1:

     (Prior to this activity, the teacher has collected and
     brought to class pictures, one of each of the following:
     food, a house, clothing, furniture, an automobile, a doctor
     and a mechanic. The teacher has also made available an
     assortment of magazines and pairs of scissors.)

     The students are seated in a semicircle, facing the bulletin
     board. The teacher begins:

          Today we are going to talk about a special
          word. The word is "consumer." A consumer
          is a person who buys things. Each of us is
          a consumer. We all buy many things. I have
          pictures of things that we buy. Look and
          listen as I name the objects in the pictures.

     The teacher places the first picture, that of food, on the
     bulletin board. The teacher continues:

          We are consumers. Consumers buy things.
          These things are called "products." These
          are some products that consumers may buy.

                              157

The teacher points to the first picture and says:

> This is a picture of food. We all buy food
> to eat. We all are consumers. Consumers are
> people who buy things. We all buy food. We
> are consumers.

The teacher continues to post the other pictures of items on the bulletin board, emphasizing that each student buys these items and, therefore, is a consumer.

After the teacher has discussed all the pictures with the students, the teacher explains:

> I am going to give each of you a magazine and
> a pair of scissors. Look through the maga-
> zine. Find a picture of something that you
> have bought or someone in your family has
> bought. Remember, a consumer is a buyer.
> You buy things. You are a consumer.

After the students have cut out pictures of items which they have purchased, the teacher remarks:

> Each of you has found a picture of something
> that you have bought. Now I want you to show
> the picture to the class and say:
>
> I am a consumer.
>
> I bought a _____.

After each student has completed the task, the teacher continues:

> You are all consumers. You have all bought
> things. We have been talking about buying
> things. But, we may also buy people's time
> and skills. If I am sick, I go to the
> doctor. Watch as I put the picture of the
> doctor on the board.

The teacher puts the picture of the doctor on the board and continues:

> If my car does not work, I go to a mechanic
> to have it fixed. I will put a picture of a
> mechanic on the board.

The teacher puts the picture of the mechanic on the board and explains:

> Now we have a picture of a doctor and a
> picture of a mechanic on the board. When
> I am sick, I go to the doctor. He helps
> me to get well. I pay him for doing this.
> I pay for his time and for what he knows.
> We call this "buying a service."

> If my car is not working, I go to the
> mechanic. I pay him to fix my car. I
> must pay him for his time. I am buying
> his service.

> Can you think of other people whose time
> and services we buy? Who can name a ser-
> vice that we buy?

After the students have named a number of people who "sell" services to the public, the teacher comments:

> You have named many people who offer their
> services to us. Consumers may buy products,
> such as cars, clothes and furniture. They
> may buy services from people, such as
> doctors and mechanics. They pay other
> people to do jobs for them. We are all
> consumers. We all buy products or services.

The activity continues until each student can demonstrate an understanding of the concept, "consumer."

MATERIALS: Chalk; chalkboard; eraser

PROCEDURE 2:

The students are seated at their desks, facing the chalkboard. The teacher explains:

    Today we are going to learn many new words.
    The first word that we will talk about is
    the word "product." I will write the word
    "product" on the board.

After the teacher has written the word on the board, he
continues:

    A product is something which is made. We
    see many products advertised on television.
    What is a product that has been advertised
    on television?

The teacher lists correct student responses under the word
"product" on the chalkboard. The teacher says:

    Many companies make products. They want to
    sell these products to us.

    Watch as I write another word on the board.
    The word is "services."

After the teacher has written the word on the board, he
comments:

    We all buy services. When we go to a dentist,
    we pay him for his time, his help and his
    knowledge. We say that the dentist offers us
    a service. We cannot fix our own teeth. We
    pay the dentist for his special skills. We
    pay for a service. Many people sell their
    services. We pay them to do special skills.
    Who can name someone else who sells his
    services?

As the students name a number of services, the teacher lists them under the word "services" on the board. Then the teacher continues:

> We will talk about one more word today. The word is "consumer." We are all consumers. I will write the word on the board.

After the teacher has written the word on the board, the teacher explains:

> A consumer is a person who buys products or services. We have already talked about the meaning of the word "product"--something that is made. We have talked about products we have seen advertised on television.
>
> We have talked about services. We pay people to work for us. They sell their special skills to us. These skills are called "services." People who buy products or services are called "consumers." We are all consumers. Let's each name a product which we have bought. Then we will each name a service we have bought. I will begin.

The teacher says:

> I am a consumer. I bought a product. The product I bought was soap. I bought a service. I paid a mechanic to fix my car.

This activity continues until each student can demonstrate an understanding of the concept, "consumer."

```
┌──────────────────────────────────────────────────────────────────────────┐
│  OBJECTIVE: Each Student Can Demonstrate an Understanding of Consumer-      │
│             related Vocabulary                                             │
└──────────────────────────────────────────────────────────────────────────┘
```

MATERIALS: 3" x 5" cards with consumer-related words, one word
             printed on each card; chalk; chalkboard; eraser

PROCEDURE 1:

    (Prior to this activity, the teacher has printed consumer-
related words on 3" x 5" index cards, one word on each
card.)

The students are seated in a semicircle, facing the chalkboard. The teacher explains:

      Today we are going to learn many new words.
      We have talked about the word "consumer."
      Remember, a consumer is a person who buys
      something. He may buy goods or services.
      We are all consumers. We all buy things.

      Today we will talk about words that con-
      sumers should know. I will write our first
      word on the board. Our first word is
      "price." Can anyone tell what the word
      "price" means?

      Tanda, what does the word "price" mean?

Tanda answers:

      "Price" is what you pay for something.

The teacher replies:

> Yes, Tanda, "price" means how much something
> costs. The price of a gallon of milk may be
> $2.00. We pay $2.00 for the milk. That is
> the price of the milk. The price is the
> amount of money we must pay for a product or
> a service. Very good, Tanda.
>
> I have written the word "price" on the
> chalkboard.

The teacher continues to introduce and to list consumer-
related vocabulary until 10 words have been discussed and
printed on the board. The teacher remarks:

> We have talked about each of the words on the
> board. There are 10 words on the board. They
> are words that are important to us as con-
> sumers. I have printed each of these 10 words
> on a card. Each of you will try to tell us
> the meaning of each of the words.
>
> Mike, you may begin. Our first word is
> "price." What is the meaning of "price"?

If Mike has difficulty defining the word, the teacher calls
on another class member to define the word. After another
class member has defined the word, Mike repeats the definition. The teacher tells Mike to hold the card with the word
"price" written on it until he has defined the remaining
vocabulary. After he has defined the other nine words, the
teacher says:

> Mike, you are holding the card with the word
> "price." Do you remember what "price" means?
> Tell us the meaning of "price."

If Mike is still unable to define the word "price," the
teacher gives additional explanation:

> Mike, "price" is what you pay for something.
> A package of gum costs 25 cents. How much do
> you pay for it? What is the price of the gum?

Mike responds:

> It is 25 cents.

The teacher remarks:

> Yes, Mike, you pay 25 cents for the package
> of gum. "Price" is the amount you pay for
> something. Now tell us the meaning of
> "price."

After Mike defines the word, the teacher comments:

> Very good, Mike. You have told us the
> meaning of all the words we have talked
> about. Now choose someone to tell us
> the meanings of the words on the board.
> You may give the cards to me.

This activity continues until each student can demonstrate
an understanding of consumer-related vocabulary.

Note: It may be necessary for the teacher to devote several
class periods to this activity. The teacher may find
it helpful to list each student's name on separate
pieces of paper. Under each student's name, the
teacher should list vocabulary words that that pupil
is unable to define.

The teacher should set aside a special time for
individual help sessions, for purposes of explanation
and drill for individual pupils. After each student
is able to understand and to define the words, his
words may be checked off the paper.

The teacher may wish to enlist the aid of parents in
helping the students.

MATERIALS: Newspapers and magazines, one of each of these for
            each student; dictionary; chalk; chalkboard; eraser

PROCEDURE 2:

The students are seated at their desks, facing the chalkboard. A newspaper and a magazine are available for each
student. The teacher explains:

> We have talked about the word "consumer." We
> know that a consumer is a person who buys
> products or services. To be a wise consumer,
> we will need to know the meaning of many con-
> sumer-related words. I want you to help me to
> find words that consumers need to know. I
> have cut an advertisement from the newspaper.
> The advertisement is for flowers for Valentine's
> Day. The ad shows two roses in a vase. It
> says "cash-and-carry." What does the phrase
> "cash-and-carry" mean?
>
> Cassandra, will you tell us what "cash-and-
> carry" means?

Cassandra responds:

> You take the flowers home after you pay for
> them.

The teacher replies:

> Yes, Cassandra, "cash-and-carry" means that a
> customer must pay for what he buys and then
> take it with him. The customer may pay by
> cash or check. He cannot have the flowers
> delivered. He must take them with him.
>
> I want each of you to look at the advertise-
> ments in the newspaper and in the magazine
> that I will give you. Find words that you
> think consumers should know. When you have
> found a word, I will write the word on the
> board. You will use the dictionary to help

166

you learn the meaning of the consumer words
you find. Some words might not be in the
dictionary. I will help you to discover the
meaning of those words.

After the students have given their consumer words to the
teacher, who lists them on the board, the teacher may wish
to make additions to the list compiled by the class.

The teacher aids and guides the students in defining consumer-related words through discussion and use of the
dictionary.

After all the words have been defined, the teacher explains:

We have talked about the meanings of all the
words on the board. Now I will give you the
definition of one of the words on the board.
Listen carefully. I will ask one of you to
tell us which word I am talking about.

The activity continues until each student is able to define
the consumer-related words.

Note: If students' reading levels impede their ability to
identify consumer vocabulary in magazine or newspaper
ads, the teacher may instruct the students to remove
ads of interest from the magazines or newspapers.
The teacher should read the ads to the students and
ask the students to recall vocabulary in the ads
which consumers will need to know.

```
┌─────────────────────────────────────────────────────────────┐
│  OBJECTIVE:  Each Student Can Verbalize Wise Shopping Habits  │
└─────────────────────────────────────────────────────────────┘
```

MATERIALS: The food section of a newspaper; coupons for food
             items; toy cash register; grocery bags; food items in
             boxes or cans; milk container with freshness date;
             trading stamps; play money; cash register receipt;
             felt-tipped marker; yarn; construction paper; paper
             punch; scissors; long table; chalk; chalkboard;
             eraser

PROCEDURE 1:

        (Prior to this activity, the teacher has collected the
        following materials: the food section of a newspaper,
        coupons for food items, toy cash register, grocery bags,
        food items in boxes or cans, milk container with freshness
        date, trading stamps, play money, cash register receipt,
        felt-tipped marker, yarn, construction paper. The teacher
        has placed these items on a table in front of the chalk-
        board.)

        The students are seated in a semicircle, facing the chalk-
        board. The teacher explains:

             Today we are going to talk about good shopping
             habits. We will talk about how to shop wisely
             at the grocery store. We will make signs that
             tell ways to shop wisely at the grocery store.
             Each of you will wear a wise shopping sign.
             When we have finished our lesson, you will be
             able to name wise shopping habits. Then we
             will tell the class next door how to shop
             wisely at the grocery.

             Let's begin. I am holding something in my
             hand. Who knows what I am holding?

                                169

Juan, tell the class what I am holding.

Juan replies:

A newspaper.

The teacher remarks:

Yes, I am holding part of a newspaper. I am
holding the food section. This part of the
paper will tell of special sales or special
values at different grocery stores. We can
look for the best buys for our money. Let's
pretend that I want to buy bread. I will
look at the newspaper to see what store has
the best price for bread. This is one way
that I might save money. This is one way to
shop wisely. I may see many foods on sale
that I will want to buy. I may go to the
store that has the lowest prices, if it is
not too far away.

Juan, how does the newspaper help me to
shop wisely?

Juan answers:

It shows the best buys. It shows how much
things cost at different stores.

The teacher comments:

Yes, Juan, we may compare prices. Now let's
make our wise shopping sign. It will say
"Use the newspaper to check prices." Place
the paper punch, a sheet of construction
paper, the scissors and the yarn in front of
you.

Now I will write the message for the sign on
the chalkboard. Copy the message on the
piece of construction paper. After you have
done that, I will punch a hole at each end

of the paper and insert a piece of yarn to
form a loop to fit around your neck. I will
tie the yarn so that you may wear the sign
around your neck.

When you have made the sign, return the yarn,
the paper punch and the scissors to the
table.

The teacher picks up several coupons and gives one to each
class member. The teacher explains:

These are coupons. They have pictures of
things which we may wish to buy. They tell
us that we may save money if we bring the
coupons to the store.

This is a coupon for toothpaste. If I bring
this coupon to the store and buy this toothpaste, I may save 12 cents. I will save
money. Who can help me make a sign about
coupons? Betty, what can we say about
coupons?

Betty replies:

"Coupons can save you money."

The teacher says:

You are correct. You can use coupons to save
money. Remember to take them to the store
with you and to give them to the person at
the register. Betty, you may make a sign to
wear that says "Coupons may save you money."

I will write "Coupons may save you money" on
the board. You may go to the table and get
a sheet of construction paper, the yarn, the
scissors and the paper punch. Write the
message on the construction paper. When you
have finished, I will help you make your
sign.

The teacher may use the props collected prior to this
activity to demonstrate the following wise buying habits:

1. Checking cash register receipts for errors.
2. Comparing prices on items such as foodstuffs.
3. Checking expiration dates on products for
    freshness.
4. Determining if accepting trading stamps is wise.
5. Watching the clerk itemizing cost of purchases
    and comparing the cost with her figures.
6. Counting change.
7. Making a list before shopping.
8. Avoiding impulse buying.
9. Returning spoiled foods.
10. Returning bottles for deposit.
11. Using recycled goods when possible.
12. Never shopping for food when you are hungry.

This activity continues until each student can verbalize
wise buying habits.

When the students and the teacher have completed making the
signs bearing wise buying suggestions and after each student
has been given a sign, the students may wear the signs to
another classroom and read the inscriptions to that class.

Note: This activity may be modified to include experiences
      in wise buying habits in other types of stores.

MATERIALS: List of several effective and ineffective shopping
             habits related to grocery buying

PROCEDURE 2:

(Prior to this activity, the teacher has made a list of
several effective and ineffective shopping habits speci-
fically related to shopping at the grocery store.)

The students are seated at their desks. The teacher
explains:

> Today we are going to talk about wise and
> unwise buying habits. I will tell you about
> the buying habits of different persons. You
> must decide if the buying habits are wise or
> unwise. You must tell the class why you feel
> as you do. Listen as I read the first account
> of buying habits.

>> Jane needs to buy chopped meat from
>> the store. She looks at the food
>> section of the newspaper to find
>> the best buys on chopped meat.

> Is Jane a shopper who uses wise shopping
> habits? John, what do you think?

John replies:

> I think Jane is a wise shopper.

The teacher asks:

> Why do you think Jane is a wise shopper?

John responds:

173

She saves money by checking prices. She
finds the best bargains.

The teacher remarks:

Yes, John, Jane is a wise shopper. She used
the newspaper to help her save time and
money.

Listen to the next statement. Does the
shopper use wise or unwise shopping habits?

Bill never bothers to count his
change.

Does Bill use wise or unwise shopping habits?
Mary, what do you think?

Mary responds:

Bill's habit is unwise. He should count his
change. The clerk might make a mistake.

The teacher agrees:

Yes, Mary, Bill's shopping habit is unwise.

When each of the students is able to differentiate between
wise and unwise shopping habits and to explain why the
habits are wise or unwise, the teacher says:

Now that we have discussed wise and unwise
shopping habits, each of you may tell the
class one wise shopping habit that we might
practice at the grocery store. Who would
like to begin?

The activity continues until each student has had the opportunity to verbalize one wise shopping habit.

OBJECTIVE: Each Student Can Demonstrate an Understanding of a Budget

MATERIALS: Large sheets of paper, one sheet for each student; crayons, nine for each student; chalk; chalkboard; eraser

PROCEDURE 1:

(Prior to this activity, the teacher has obtained large sheets of paper, one sheet for each student, and crayons, nine for each student.)

The students are seated at their desks, facing the chalkboard. The teacher explains:

Today we are going to talk about the word "budget." Sometimes you hear parents talk about a budget. A budget might be thought of as a plan. Let's talk about Mr. Jones. Mr. Jones has a budget. Mr. Jones has a job. He is paid once a month. During every month, Mr. Jones has certain bills to pay. These bills might be called expenses. Who can name some bills that Mr. Jones must pay every month? I will write the expenses on the board after you name them.

Lee, what is one bill or expense that Mr. Jones has every month?

Lee replies:

Food.

The teacher remarks:

> Yes, Lee, Mr. Jones must buy food every
> month. What other bills or expenses does
> Mr. Jones have every month?

The teacher continues to list fixed expenses on the board,
as the students name them. After the teacher has listed all
the fixed expenses that the students can think of, he introduces other items, such as savings, entertainment, miscellaneous items, that should be included in a budget. In all,
the teacher lists nine items on the board.

The teacher then draws a circle on the board, explaining how
much of Mr. Jones' salary is spent for each item listed on
the board. The teacher explains:

> Now you know how Mr. Jones spends his money.
> When you earn money, you will want to make a
> budget like Mr. Jones did.
>
> I am going to give each of you a piece of
> paper and some crayons. Each of you is going
> to make a budget. You do not know how much
> money you will make, so you will draw a circle
> and just put in your expenses. The expenses
> are listed on the board if you need to refer
> to them.
>
> First, draw a big circle on your paper. Watch
> me draw a circle on the board.

The teacher demonstrates by drawing a circle for the
students. Then he explains:

> You must divide your circle into parts. Each
> of you will need nine parts in your circle.
> The first part will be for the expense of
> housing. It will be the biggest part of the
> circle. You will probably spend most of your
> money on housing.

The teacher divides the circle on the board into nine per-
centage parts and labels each one. The teacher instructs
the students to print the name of each expense on its

corresponding part of the circle, using a different colored crayon for each expense.

After the circles have been completed, the teacher comments:

> Now each of you has made a budget circle. You can see what part of your money goes for each expense. When you begin to earn money and to pay bills, you may use your budget to help you plan how you will spend your money.

The activity continues until each student can demonstrate an understanding of what a budget is and of how to make one.

Note: Circle divisions indicate food; clothing; rent; utilities; savings; medical, dental, recreational and miscellaneous spending.

MATERIALS: One box of legal-size envelopes; felt-tipped pen;
             play money; chalk; chalkboard; eraser

PROCEDURE 2:

   (Prior to this activity, the teacher, using a felt-tipped
   pen, has printed the name of each fixed expense on an
   envelope.)

   The students are seated at their desks, facing the chalkboard.
   The teacher begins:

        Today we are going to talk about budgets. A
        budget might be thought of as a plan. A per-
        son knows how much money he will make each
        month. A person must plan how he will spend
        his money. Some expenses are called "fixed
        expenses." These bills come due each month.
        Can you name some bills that come due every
        month?

        Melvin, what are some of these fixed expenses?

   Melvin responds:

        They are rent and food.

   The teacher replies:

        Very good, Melvin. You have named two fixed
        expenses. Who can name other bills that
        occur each month?

   As the students name the various fixed expenses, the teacher
   lists them on the board. After the list has been completed,
   the teacher reads the list to the class. The teacher comments:

        We have listed all our fixed expenses. We
        have other expenses which might not come each
        month. We must still set aside money for

178

these expenses, just in case we need it. We
must plan to set aside money for savings,
recreation, medical expenses, emergency expenses, insurance and odds and ends. We
call these "miscellaneous expenses."

Now we can see where our money will be
going. We are going to work on a budget
plan for Mr. Jones. Mr. Jones takes home
$630.00 a month. He makes more money, but
his employer takes out money for retirement,
social security, income tax and health insurance. Mr. Jones is left with $630.00 to
take home.

I have printed the name of each expense in
our budget on an envelope. We have $630.00
in play money. Let's look at our first
expense. It is rent. Mr. Jones pays $175.00
for rent. I will write $175.00 on the en-
velope marked "rent." Now I will count out
$175.00 from Mr. Jones' $630.00 take-home
pay. John, put this $175.00 in the envelope
marked "rent." Mr. Jones has $455.00 left
after paying rent.

After John has placed $175.00 of play money in the envelope
marked "rent," the teacher continues the activity until each
fixed expense in the budget has been covered. The teacher
says:

We have accounted for all of Mr. Jones' fixed
expenses. We have $70.00 left for Mr. Jones'
other expenses: savings, recreation, medical
expenses and others.

We may divide this money among the budget
items that are left. How much do you think
Mr. Jones can spend for recreation?

The students decide upon reasonable ways to divide Mr. Jones'
money into the categories which remain. After they have
accounted for all the money and after the teacher has placed
the play money in the proper envelopes, the teacher concludes:

179

Now we know how Mr. Jones spends the money
that he earns. When each of you earns a
salary or a wage, you will need to make your
own budget. Each of you will have a different
budget. You will spend the money which you
earn in different ways. You will have different expenses, but you will still need a
plan for spending your money. We call this
plan or schedule a budget.

The activity continues, with the teacher using other budget
plans, until each student is able to demonstrate an understanding of what a budget is and of how to make one.

Note: The teacher should review vocabulary words with the
        students. These words should include "budget,"
        "income," "salary," "wage," "social security,"
        "retirement," "deductions," "fixed expenses,"
        "schedule."

MATERIALS: Large six-part figure of a person; bulletin board;
         thumbtacks; chalk; chalkboard; eraser

PROCEDURE 1:

   (Prior to this activity, the teacher has made a figure of a
   person, large enough to be viewed easily by the class members
   when it is placed on the bulletin board. The figure consists
   of six parts: the head which is circular in shape; the trunk
   which is rectangular; the arms which are rectangular; and the
   feet which are triangular. The following phrases have been
   printed by the teacher on the body of the figure, one on each
   part of the body: "Have good shopping habits"; "teach others";
   "share with others"; "do not waste"; "pay your bills";
   "speak out.")

   The students are seated at their desks, facing the bulletin
   board and the chalkboard. The teacher places the figure on
   the bulletin board and says:

      We have talked about the word "consumer." A
      consumer is a person who buys products or
      services. We are all consumers. We have
      also talked about the word "responsibility."
      We must be responsible consumers.

      Today we will talk about ways we might be
      responsible consumers. I have placed a
      figure of a person on the board. We will
      pretend that it is a consumer. On each part
      of the person's body, I have written phrases.

These phrases will help us to remember ways
that we might be responsible consumers.

Look at the head. On the head I have written
the words "have good shopping habits." Who
can think of ways that a consumer might practice good shopping habits?

Maureen, what are some good shopping habits?

Maureen answers:

Count your change.

The teacher replies:

Yes, Maureen, a wise consumer will count his
change. I will write your answer on the
board. Who can name other good shopping
habits?

The teacher lists responses of the students on the chalkboard. After a number of suggestions have been listed,
the teacher explains:

We have talked about one of the responsibilities of a consumer, to have good
shopping habits. We have named many ways
that we can be wise shoppers. Listen as I
name them.

The teacher reads the suggestions written on the board and
suggests additional ways that consumers might practice wise
shopping habits.

The teacher explains:

Now we will talk about another responsibility
of a consumer. Look at the figure on the
board. The words on the body of the figure
say "teach others." We are responsible for
teaching others how to be responsible consumers. We might teach friends, family,

neighbors or our own children how to be
responsible consumers. Who can tell us a
way that we might teach others to be responsible consumers?

Tom, can you help us?

Tom responds:

I would tell mothers and fathers not to buy
toys with sharp parts for their little
children.

The teacher replies:

Yes, Tom, that is one way that we might teach
others to be responsible consumers. I will
write your idea on the board.

After each student has named a way in which he might educate
others as to their responsibilities as consumers, the teacher
reads the suggestions listed on the board and offers additional ones to the class.

This activity continues until each of the six areas of consumer responsibility printed on the figure has been dis-
cussed--"have good shopping habits"; "teach others"; "share
with others"; "do not waste"; "pay your bills"; "speak out";
and until each student is able to demonstrate an understanding
of the responsibilities of a consumer.

<u>MATERIALS</u>: Chalk; chalkboard; eraser; paper, one sheet for each
              student; pencils, one pencil for each student; stapler

<u>PROCEDURE 2</u>:

    (Prior to this activity, the teacher has written the following
    sentences on the chalkboard:

        1. I will practice wise shopping habits.
        2. I will teach my family members how to be
            wise consumers.
        3. I will not be fooled by false ads.
        4. I will be responsible for my debts.
        5. I will know where to go to seek help for
            products or services that are poor.)

The students are seated at their desks, facing the chalkboard. The teacher explains:

    Today we are going to talk about ways that we
    might be more responsible consumers. I have
    written some ways that we might be responsible
    consumers on the board. Listen as I read the
    sentences on the board.

After the teacher has read the sentences to the class, he
continues:

    These are things that a consumer might do to
    demonstrate responsibility. You are going to
    form groups. There will be three people in
    each group. Each group will be assigned one
    of the topics on the board. Mary, Lee and
    Bess may be in the first group. They will
    find ways that a consumer could practice wise
    shopping habits. They will write their ideas
    on paper that I will give them. When they
    are finished, they will read their suggestions
    to the class. The class may wish to add ideas
    to the list.

    When all the groups are finished, we will put
    our ideas together. We will make a booklet

184

for the library. Other students will be able
to read our booklet and to learn how to be
responsible consumers.

Now I will assign you to groups. I will give
each group one of the topics on the board. I
will give each group paper and pencils.

You may begin to work in your group as soon
as you receive your paper and pencil. I will
come to each group to offer suggestions, to
answer questions and to help with problems.
You may begin. In 20 minutes, you should
have completed your assignment.

The teacher assists the members of each group in formulating
ideas about ways in which they might demonstrate consumer
responsibility related to the topics assigned.

After the members of each group have completed their assignment and have read their suggestions, the teacher encourages
the other class members to make additional suggestions as to
how consumer responsibility may be exercised in relation to
each topic.

After the additional suggestions have been formulated in
writing by the groups, the teacher comments:

Now I will collect the papers from each of the
groups. I will place the sheets of paper between two pieces of construction paper. I
will write the name of our booklet on one of
the pieces of construction paper. The name
of our booklet is "How to Be a Responsible
Consumer." I will place the other piece of
construction paper behind your comment pages.
I will staple the papers together to form a
booklet.

After the booklet has been completed, the class should offer
it to the librarian, requesting that it be made available to
all students.

MATERIALS: Advertisements without descriptions; advertisements
with descriptions; chalk; chalkboard; eraser

PROCEDURE 1:

(Prior to this activity, the teacher has collected and
brought to class several advertisements which show products
and use descriptive words in telling about the products.
The teacher also has brought pictures of products, without
written descriptions, one picture for each student.)

The students are seated at their desks, facing the chalkboard. The teacher explains:

> Today we are going to look at some pictures
> of products. Remember, a product is something
> that we may buy. We are going to describe,
> or tell about, products. I will put a picture
> of the first product on the board.
>
> What is the product, John?

John replies:

> It is a towel.

The teacher remarks:

> Very good, John. The product pictured in
> this advertisement is a towel. I will read

187

the advertisement to you. Remember to listen
for descriptive words. When I have finished
reading, I will ask you to tell me some of
the descriptive words in the advertisement.

The teacher reads the advertisement aloud to the class and
then asks:

Who can name some of the descriptive words
in the advertisement? I will write the words
on the board.

Craig, please tell us some of the descriptive
words.

Craig responds:

One is "thick." Another is "big."

The teacher lists the descriptive words on the board and
remarks:

We have listed descriptive words on the board.
These words describe the towel in the advertisement. Listen as I read the words to you.
If you want me to tell the meaning of any of
the words, raise your hand.

The teacher reads the descriptive words to the class. Then
he explains:

Now we will look at another advertisement.
The product is lipstick. Listen for the
descriptive words in the advertisement. I
will ask someone to name the descriptive words
for us. I will list the words on the board.

After the students have been able to list descriptive words
from several advertisements and after the teacher has listed
these descriptive words on the board, the teacher continues:

We have found many descriptive words. These
words tell about or describe the products we
have seen in the advertisements. I am going
to give each of you a picture of a product.
You may name descriptive words you would use
to tell about your product. Maybe one of the
words on the board could be used to describe
your product. Raise your hand when you are
ready.

After several students have raised their hands, the teacher
says:

Marcy, your product is candy. What descriptive words would you use to tell about the
candy?

Marcy replies:

Candy is "sweet." Candy is "delicious."

The teacher comments:

Very good, Marcy. You have described your
product, candy. Now I will read the words on
the board. Let's see if any of the words on
the board might be used to describe candy.

This activity continues until each student is able to
describe a product.

MATERIALS: Approximately 20 to 25 pictures of products advertised
             in magazines; bulletin board; thumbtacks; chalk;
             chalkboard; eraser

PROCEDURE 2:

(Prior to this activity, the teacher has collected 20 to 25
pictures of products advertised in magazines and has posted
5 of these pictures on the bulletin board.)

The students are seated at their desks, facing the bulletin
board. The teacher explains:

> Today we are going to describe products. Re-
> member, a product is something that we might
> buy. We have talked about products in other
> lessons. I have placed five pictures of
> products on the board. I am going to describe
> one of the products on the board. Remember,
> "to describe" means "to tell about." I want
> you to listen to the description. Raise your
> hand when you can tell which product I am
> describing.

The teacher describes one of the pictures of products posted
on the bulletin board. After the teacher has described the
product, he selects a student to identify the product
described.

If the student is unable to select the product described,
the teacher gives additional explanation:

> I will repeat the description and will add
> additional words to describe the product.
> After I have told you more about the product,
> you may have another chance to identify it.

The teacher then describes the product, giving additional
descriptive words.

If the student selects the product described, the teacher
says:

Very good. You know that I have described
the towel. I used the words "thick,"
"thirsty," "soft," "absorbent," and "pastel-
colored" to describe the picture of the
towel. Who can tell us other descriptive
words that I might have used?

The teacher lists on the chalkboard additional descriptive
words given by the students.

After all the pictures of products on the bulletin board
have been described by the teacher and identified by the
students, the teacher explains:

You have identified all the products which I
have described. You have used additional
words to describe the products in the pictures
on the board. Now I will give each of you a
picture of a product.

Each of you may show your product to the class
and use descriptive words in sentences when
telling about your product. You will make up
your own advertisement for the product. When
you have prepared your advertisement, which
will describe your product, raise your hand.

This activity continues until each student is able to
describe a product.

MATERIALS: Desk; chair

PROCEDURE 1:

The students and the teacher are seated in a semicircle,
leaving an acting area large enough for a desk and a chair.
The teacher explains:

Today we are going to learn what to do when
we have a problem when we are shopping.

I will tell stories about different consumers.
Each of these consumers will have a problem.
I will ask you to tell how you would help
each of these consumers solve his problem.

Our first consumer's name is Sandra. Sandra
went to the supermarket. Her mother asked
her to buy a box of crackers for 49 cents.
Sandra knew she would get 51 cents change
back from her dollar. The checkout person
did not give her the correct change. What
should Sandra do?

Ann, please come here. I will be the checkout person. You will be Sandra. We will act
out what happened. You will act out what you
would do to solve the problem.

When Ann and the teacher have completed the role playing by
solving the problem, the teacher continues this activity.

Other problems to be solved might include losing a wallet, exchanging a sweater that has a defect; returning a carton of sour milk; asking for an advertised special.

This activity continues until each student is able to role play a situation in which a consumer-related problem is solved.

<u>MATERIALS</u>: Desk; two chairs

<u>PROCEDURE 2</u>:

   The students and the teacher are seated in a semicircle,
   leaving an acting area large enough for a desk and two
   chairs. The teacher divides the class members into two
   teams and explains:

          You have learned many things about buying
          products. You know how to shop wisely for
          products for yourselves and for your homes.
          Today you will learn what to do when the
          products you buy are bad or when there are
          mistakes in the bills you must pay. I will
          assign two students on both teams the same
          problem to role play. The other team members
          may help them prepare their solutions to the
          problem. Both teams will have five minutes
          to prepare their solutions. After the as-
          signed students have acted out their teams'
          solutions, we will decide which team has
          solved the problem in the best way.

   After the five minutes has elapsed, the teacher calls the
   two selected students from the first team up to the desk and
   chairs to role play the problem and their solution to it.
   When they have completed their role playing, the two members
   selected from the opposing team role play the problem and
   their solution to it. After they have finished, the class
   members discuss the solutions and decide which one is the
   best.

   The teacher then assigns another consumer-related problem
   to two other members from both teams.

   This activity continues until each student is able to role
   play a situation in which a consumer-related problem is
   solved.

SECTION **5**

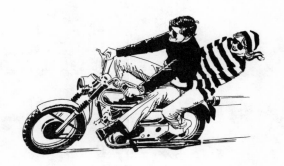

I Am a Traveler

TRAVEL-RELATED VOCABULARY

arrival time
avenue
backpack
boulevard
cable car
cancelled
caution
commuter
courtesy
delay
departure
destination
detour
escalator
gear
highway
hike
insurance
interstate
laws
license
lifeboat
life preserver
luggage

mechanic
merge
motel
overpass
path
radar
regulations
reservations
road signs
safety
schedule
speed
stopover
storm warnings
street
subway
terminal
trail
transfer
traveler
tunnel
van
vehicle
visa

| OBJECTIVE: | Each Student Can Demonstrate an Understanding of the Concept, "Travel" |

MATERIALS: Envelope containing several pictures of places students would like to visit; the words, "how," "where," "why," printed on cardboard strips, one word per strip; sheets of paper; felt-tipped pen; bulletin board; thumbtacks

PROCEDURE 1:

(Prior to this activity, the teacher has printed the words, "how," "where," "why," in large print on strips of cardboard, one word per strip. He has also gathered up pictures of places the students might be interested in visiting and has placed these pictures in a large envelope.)

The students are seated in a semicircle, facing the bulletin board. The teacher places a large envelope on the bulletin board. The teacher begins:

> Today we are going to talk about the word "travel." What does it mean to travel? What do you do when you travel?
>
> Jill, what does it mean to travel?

Jill responds:

> It means "to walk." It means "to go somewhere."

The teacher agrees:

> Yes, Jill, when we travel, we go from place
> to place. There are many ways to travel. I
> will put the cardboard strip with the word
> "how" on the bulletin board. I would like
> each of you to think of ways that you might
> travel. I will write these ways down on
> paper.
>
> Ted, what is one way that you might travel?

Ted answers:

> I can travel by bus.

The teacher agrees:

> Yes, you can travel by bus.

After students have named several methods of travel and
after the teacher has recorded their responses on paper, the
teacher places the paper under the "how" on the bulletin
board. The teacher may then bring unusual methods of travel
to the attention of the students.

Once the students are aware of the many different methods of
travel, the teacher places the cardboard strip bearing the
word "where" on the board. The teacher explains:

> I have placed the word "where" on the board.
> When you travel, you are usually trying to
> get to a special place. You might be
> traveling to the library, or you might be
> traveling to Disney World. The special place
> to go is your destination.
>
> I will give each of you a picture of some-
> place that you would like to visit. Joan, I
> will give you the first picture. What is the
> special place in your picture?

Joan responds:

   It is Disney World.

The teacher asks:

   Have you traveled to Disney World?

Joan answers:

   Yes!

The teacher comments:

   Let's pretend that you are going to travel to
   Disney World again. Look at the word "how"
   on the board. How would you like to travel
   to Disney World?

Joan answers:

   I would drive.

The teacher remarks.

   Yes, you could drive to Disney World. You
   would not walk. It is too far. You could
   also fly or take a special bus there.

   You have told how you would travel. You have
   also told where you would travel. Now I will
   place the word "why" on the board.

   Joan, why would you travel to Disney World?

Joan answers:

It is fun to see all the rides. I like to go
on trips.

The teacher comments:

Joan has told us why she wants to travel to
Disney World. She wants to see the rides,
and she likes to travel. She may also learn
many new things while she is traveling. She
may meet new people.

There are many reasons to travel. Sometimes
we might travel to a different city to find
a better job. We might travel to visit relatives. I will write some reasons why we
travel on the sheet of paper under the word
"why" on the board.

We have told what the word "travel" means.
We have talked about how we might travel.
We have talked about where we might travel.
We have talked about why we might travel.

Who would like to choose another picture?
Remember, try to tell where you are going to
travel, why you would like to travel there
and how you would travel to the place in the
picture.

The teacher assists each student in developing the "how,"
"where," "why" of travel. Each student's response as to
mode of travel, destination and motivation for travel is
listed on paper under the proper category on the bulletin
board.

This activity continues until each student is able to
demonstrate an understanding of the concept, "travel."

<u>MATERIALS</u>: Chalkboard; chalk; eraser

<u>PROCEDURE</u> <u>2</u>:

The students are seated at their desks, facing the chalkboard. The teacher has written the following definition on
the board:

      _____ means "to go from place to place;
    to walk or to run; to move or to pass."

The teacher explains:

    I have written a definition on the board.
    Remember, to define a word is to tell what
    the word means. Listen as I read the de-
    finition. Who can tell the word that is
    being defined?

    Larry, what word am I defining?

If Larry cannot supply the word "travel," the teacher
explains:

    Larry, I am defining the word "travel."
    "Travel" means "to go from place to place;
    to walk or to run; to move or to pass."
    Now I will repeat the definition. Tell us
    the word that is being defined.

If Larry can provide the word "travel," the teacher
responds:

    Yes, Larry, I am defining the word "travel."

The teacher then reads the definition aloud to the class,
supplying the missing word and writing the word in the blank
on the chalkboard. The teacher says:

Today we are going to talk about traveling.
We will talk about ways that we might travel.
We will talk about reasons that we might
travel. We will talk about how traveling
might help us in unexpected ways. I will
write the words "how," "why," "benefits,"
on the board.

Let's look at the word "how" first. You
may tell us as many ways to travel as you
can.

On the board the teacher lists methods of travel named by
the students. After all student responses have been listed,
the teacher may wish to add unusual methods of travel not
mentioned by the students. The teacher should define and
reinforce new vocabulary. The teacher says:

We have named many ways to travel. Now let's
think of reasons why people travel. As you
name them, I will write the reasons on the
board.

After the students have volunteered a number of reasons for
traveling, the teacher may wish to supply additional reasons,
which he lists on the board. The teacher continues:

Let's think of ways we could benefit from
traveling. I will list these on the board
under the word "benefit," as you name them.

After the students have volunteered a number of benefits of
travel, the teacher may wish to supply additional benefits
of travel, which he lists on the board. The teacher comments:

Now we can see how we might travel, why we
might travel and what the benefits of travel
are. Let's talk about Mr. Jones' trip. Look
at the word "how" on the board. Mr. Jones
wants to take a trip to Japan. How might Mr.
Jones travel?

After the students have selected the best means of transportation, the teacher says:

204

I will tell you why Mr. Jones is traveling to
Japan. He is traveling to Japan to begin a
new job. What do you think are some benefits
that Mr. Jones might experience from his
travels?

After the students have given a number of benefits associated
with travel, the teacher encourages them to recall trips that
they have made and to tell how they traveled, why they
traveled and what benefits they derived from their travels.

This activity continues until each student can demonstrate
an understanding of the concept, "travel."

OBJECTIVE: **Each Student Can Demonstrate an Understanding of Travel-related Vocabulary**

MATERIALS: Travel-related vocabulary list; chalk; chalkboard; eraser

PROCEDURE 1:

The students are seated at their desks, facing the chalkboard. The teacher explains:

> Today we are going to learn more about traveling. We have talked about what the word "travel" means. We have talked about how we might travel, where we might travel and why we travel. We know that travel means "to go from place to place." We know that a traveler is a person who goes from place to place.
>
> Today we will talk about words that travelers will need to know. I will write the words on the board. I will tell you what the words mean. You will learn many new words today. Listen carefully. I am going to write the word "highway" on the board.

After the teacher has written the word on the board, the teacher remarks:

> This word is "highway." A highway is a road. It is a main road. Many cars travel on the

207

highway. If you are a licensed driver, you
may drive on the highway.

Rose, please tell us what a highway is.

Rose responds:

It is a road.

The teacher agrees:

Yes, Rose, a highway is a road. It is a main
road. Many trucks and automobiles are driven
on the highway. Well done.

The teacher continues to add, define and reinforce vocabulary
related to travel until the number of words on the board is
equal to the number of students in the class. The teacher
says:

There are ____ travel words on the board. I
will point to each word as I read it.

After the teacher has read the words, he continues:

Now I will talk about one of the words written
on the board. Listen as I define one of the
words. Can you tell us which word I am
talking about? If you can, raise your hand.

This word means a road. It is a main road.
Many cars and trucks travel on this road.
Listen as I read the words on the board.
Which word means a main road?

Ralph, which word means a main road?

Ralph answers:

It is "highway."

The teacher says:

       Very good, Ralph. A highway is a main road.
       You are correct.

After the students have associated all the words written on the board with their definitions, the teacher introduces 10 new vocabulary terms, defines the words and aids the students in matching the definitions given to the words written on the board.

This activity continues until each student can demonstrate an understanding of vocabulary related to travel.

MATERIALS: Travel-related vocabulary lists; chalk; chalkboard;
             eraser

PROCEDURE 2:

The students are seated at their desks, facing the chalkboard. The teacher explains:

> Today we are going to talk about words that
> travelers should know. We are going to define
> these words. Remember, "to define" means "to
> tell what the word means." I will write the
> first word on the board. Watch as I write
> the word. The word is "traveler."

The teacher writes the word on the board and says:

> A traveler is a person who travels. A
> traveler is a person who moves from place
> to place.

The teacher continues to write vocabulary words on the
board, to define and to discuss the words until there are
as many words on the board as there are students in the
class. After all the words on the board have been defined,
the teacher remarks:

> We have talked about the words on the board.
> John, look at the first word on the board.
> The word is "traveler." Can you define the
> word for the class? What does the word mean?

John responds:

> A traveler is a person who goes from place
> to place.

The teacher replies:

Very good, John. A traveler is a person who
moves from place to place.

This activity continues until each student can demonstrate
an understanding of travel-related vocabulary.

Note: It will take several class periods to complete the
        objective. A list of suggested vocabulary is provided
        on page 196. The teacher may add vocabulary to this
        list or delete inappropriate terms.

MATERIALS: Six 8½" x 5½" cards, each card containing a question
from Procedure 1; bulletin board; thumbtacks

PROCEDURE 1:

The students are seated in a semicircle, facing the bulletin
board. The teacher places the six question cards on the
bulletin board and explains:

> We have talked about traveling and about trips
> we have taken. Today we will organize all our
> ideas so that each of you will be able to tell
> about a trip. These cards I have made will
> help you to remember your trip. Listen as I
> tell you what is written on each card.

The teacher reads the questions on each of the six cards.
These questions are listed below:

1. Where did I go?
2. How did I get there?
3. What did I see?
4. Who was with me?
5. What did I enjoy about my trip?
6. What did I learn?

The teacher continues:

> If you can answer all the questions, you will
> be able to tell a story about your travels.

213

Think of a trip you have taken. Be ready to
tell us about your trip.

When the students are ready to discuss their trips, the
teacher says:

Rose, you may begin. Please answer the
questions on each of the six cards. Be sure
to use sentences.

If Rose cannot answer the questions, the teacher says:

Rose, you need help in telling about your
trip. I will write the questions on a sheet
of paper. Ask your parents to help you
write the answers to the questions on the
sheet of paper. We will discuss your trip
after you return the paper.

If Rose answers the questions on each of the six cards in
describing her trip, the teacher praises her and selects
another student to discuss his trip.

Note: To increase the difficulty of the task, the teacher
may remove the cards and have the students tell of a
travel experience in sequential sentences without the
aid of the cue cards.

If the students' parents are not responsive, the
teacher may wish to modify the assignment, allowing
students to tell of a trip that they would enjoy
taking. He could easily modify questions to accomplish this task.

<u>MATERIALS</u>: Mimeographed sheets, containing questions used in
Procedure 2; one sheet for each student

<u>PROCEDURE 2</u>:

(Prior to this activity, the teacher and the students have
compiled a list of questions relevant to travel. The teacher
has written the students' responses on a ditto master and has
duplicated copies for the class members.)

The students are seated at their desks. The teacher dis-
tributes a copy of the compiled questions to each student.
The teacher reads the questions which should include:
"Where did I go?" "When did I go?" "What did I like?"
"What did I learn?"

The teacher instructs the students to recall a trip they have
taken. (If students have difficulty in recalling a specific
trip, the teacher should remind them of field trips taken by
the class.) The teacher explains:

We are going to tell about our travels. Look
at the questions written on your paper. Use
the questions to help you tell about your
trip. You might not answer all the questions.
You might want to add more information in
telling about your trip.

After one student has related his travel experience, the
teacher continues:

Look at the list of questions. Put a check
next to each question that the speaker answered in his talk.

When each student has marked the questions that were answered
in the speaker's talk, the teacher remarks:

John, read the list of questions that you
think Susan answered in her speech.

After John has read the list, the teacher continues:

215

John, you are a good listener. You checked
all the questions that Susan answered in her
talk.

This activity continues until each student has had the opportunity to verbalize a travel experience.

Note: The checklist will help the students to develop
listening skills and will help them to sequence their
own information.

The teacher might arrange special trips, for example,
a trip to a courthouse, one to a health department,
one to a vocational center. During the trips, the
teacher should take slides so that the students may
use the slide-projected pictures to plan a travelogue,
thus helping develop their language skills.

```
┌──────────────────────────────────────────────────────────────────┐
│  OBJECTIVE: Each Student Can Demonstrate an Understanding of Procedures │
│             Necessary for Planning a Trip                          │
└──────────────────────────────────────────────────────────────────┘
```

MATERIALS: Three teacher-made cards: "How Will We Get There?,"
             "What Will We Eat?," "What Will We Do?"; paper, one
             sheet for each student; pencils, one pencil for each
             student

PROCEDURE 1:

    (Prior to this activity, the teacher has printed the words
    "How Will We Get There?" on one card, the words "What Will
    We Eat?" on another and the words "What Will We Do?" on a
    third.)

    The students are seated in three groups. The teacher
    remarks:

        We have learned many things about traveling.
        Today we are going to plan a trip that we may
        all take. Next Saturday we will go to DeSoto
        Park. We will leave at 10:00 a.m. We will
        return at 6:30 p.m. We must plan our trip
        carefully.

    The teacher holds up the first card and explains:

        The first cards says "How Will We Get There?"
        The first group may take this card. Think of
        the best way we can get to DeSoto Park. It
        may be by bus, by foot, by car or by van.
        You will decide the best way for the class to
        go.

                            217

The second card says "What Will We Eat?" The second group may decide what foods to bring and who will bring them. Remember, we will be at the park for eight hours. We will need snacks, drinks and lunch.

The third card says "What Will We Do?" We will need many games. Group Three may decide what we will do at the park.

All the groups may now make their plans.

The students work in groups, writing down their plans for the day at the park. The teacher observes each group, offering advice and suggestions if necessary.

When the groups have completed their assignments, the teacher asks each group's members to report on what they have planned.

This activity continues until each student is able to demonstrate the ability to help plan a trip.

MATERIALS: Paper, one sheet for each student; pencils, one pencil
            for each student; chalk; chalkboard; eraser

PROCEDURE 2:

    The students are seated in four groups. The teacher explains:

> Today we are going to plan a class trip to
> Disney World. Group One members will be
> responsible for determining what items class
> members should pack for the trip. They will
> tell the number and types of suitcases to
> take on the trip.
>
> Group Two members will estimate how much the
> trip will cost. They will suggest ways that
> we might raise money for the trip. They will
> need to know that we will be traveling in
> three cars and that we will be staying for
> one night in a motel. This group will need
> to plan a budget for food, entertainment,
> lodging and transportation costs. They will
> need to talk with members of groups Three
> and Four to aid them in estimating the cost
> of our trip.
>
> Group Three members will take the road map
> and find out how long it will take to drive to
> Disney World. They should go to Mr. Jones,
> the driver education teacher, who will help
> them find out the cost of gasoline for the
> trip. He will talk to them about what safety
> measures are necessary for car travel.
>
> Group Four members will take hotel and motel
> brochures and find the best place for us to
> stay. Remember, we will be spending one
> night in a motel. Some places may have
> special rates for school groups.

The teacher circulates among the groups, helping as necessary. When the groups have completed their assignments, the
teacher asks each group to report to the class. As each
group reports, the teacher writes pertinent information on
the chalkboard.

This activity continues until each student is able to demonstrate an understanding of procedures necessary for planning a trip.

MATERIALS: Sets of clothing and accessory pictures, none of
which are identical, one set for each student; pictures of different climate areas; suitcase

PROCEDURE 1:

(Prior to this activity the teacher has collected sets of
clothing and accessory pictures and pictures of two different
climate areas. Each set of pictures consists of 10 articles
of clothing or accessories for different climates and occa-
sions.)

The students are seated at their desks. The teacher gives
each student a set of clothing and accessory pictures and
explains:

Today we are going to talk about trips to different places. You will decide what you would
take in your suitcase if you were going to
travel to these places. Listen carefully as I
tell you about the first trip.

The teacher holds up a picture of the first vacation area
and continues:

The first trip is to Clearwater Beach in
Florida in June. It is hot during this time
of the year in Florida. You will be staying
a week. You will want to fish and to swim.

221

You will not be going to any fancy places.
You will be going to bed early.

Now look at your pictures. Who has a picture
of something that would be needed on this
trip? If you have something we should pack
for the trip, raise your hand. If you are
correct, you may place the item in this suitcase.

After the teacher and the students have packed appropriate
items for traveling to this vacation spot, the teacher
continues:

We have packed sunglasses, sun lotion, fishing
poles, slacks, water skis, shirts, underwear,
socks, sandals, shoes and many other items.
They are all needed for our trip to Florida.

Why didn't we pack an overcoat?

The teacher calls on a student to explain why this article
of clothing would be inappropriate for the Florida trip.

The teacher collects the remaining pictures from the students
and removes the other pictures from the suitcase. He distributes new sets of clothing and accessory pictures to the
students. The teacher introduces the second vacation area
and shows the students a picture of it.

This activity continues until each student can classify items
appropriate to particular vacation areas.

MATERIALS: Three filmstrips, one filmstrip of San Francisco, one
of Grand Teton National Park, one of Key West, Florida;
five pictures of suitcases, each picture of a different
suitcase, or five actual suitcases; film projector;
screen; copies of local newspaper, one copy for each
student

PROCEDURE 2:

The students are seated in a semicircle, facing the screen.
The teacher explains:

When we travel, we must know what to pack. I
have filmstrips of three different places in
the United States. We will look at the filmstrip of San Francisco first. John, please
turn out the lights.

After John has turned out the lights, the teacher explains:

This filmstrip shows San Francisco. San
Francisco is a city in California. We will
plan to pack for a three-day trip to San
Francisco.

The teacher proceeds to show the filmstrip, emphasizing
climate, places to visit, things to see and do. After the
teacher has completed showing the filmstrip, the students
decide where they would like to visit in San Francisco and
in what activities they would like to participate.

The teacher continues:

We know we will spend three days in San
Francisco. We can look in the newspaper and
see what the temperature is in the city.

The teacher gives each student a copy of the newspaper and
remarks:

Turn to page 2. See the National Weather
Guide. What is the temperature in San
Francisco?

After the students have found the temperature of San Francisco
in the National Weather Guide, the teacher says:

Now we know the temperature, we know where we
are going, what we will be doing and how long
we will be staying. What should we pack?

Students' answers might include a pair of slacks, comfortable
tops, comfortable shoes, dress outfit, dress shoes, socks or
panty hose, sets of underclothes, pajamas, raincoat or
sweater coat, camera, deodorant, toothpaste, toothbrush,
jewelry.

After the teacher has discussed the value of wash-and-wear
clothing with the students, he shows the students the pictures
of the suitcases (or the actual suitcases) and asks the
students to select one that would be appropriate to use. He
reminds the students that they should not burden themselves
with excess weight.

The teacher then shows slides of Grand Teton National Park
and repeats the procedure of having the students find the
temperature in the newspaper. He emphasizes that this type
of trip will require more rugged clothing than the trip to
San Francisco. He explains that activities might include
hiking, riding horses, rubber rafting the rapids, camping,
etc. The students then decide what type of clothing to pack
for this trip and what type of suitcase to take. Their
answers should include sleeping bags, back packs, insect
repellant, sun lotion, jeans, boots, sweaters, jackets,
ponchos.

The teacher then shows the slides of Key West, introduces
another type of vacation, and repeats the procedure of
having the students find the temperature in the newspaper.
The students again are asked to decide what type of clothing
to pack--bathing suits, terri robes, sandals, shorts, light
clothing, sunglasses, fishing rods and what type of suitcase
to take. The teacher and students discuss the advisability
of bringing heavy equipment, such as scuba diving gear and
wet suits, or of renting such equipment.

This activity continues until each student has had the opportunity to list appropriate items to take on different
types of trips.

OBJECTIVE: **Each Student Can Verbalize Solutions to Problems That Might Be Experienced While He Is Traveling**

MATERIALS: Chalk; chalkboard; eraser

PROCEDURE 1:

(Prior to this activity, the teacher has thought up several stories involving travel problems.)

The students are seated in a semicircle, facing the chalkboard. The teacher explains:

We have learned many things about traveling. Today we are going to talk about problems we may have while we are traveling. We will talk about ways that we may solve these problems. I am going to tell you a story. It is a travel story. Travelers in the story have a problem. Listen to the story. See if you can help to solve the problem.

The teacher tells the first travel story:

John and his family have taken a trip to Disney World. It is Saturday. It is noon. John and his family have waited in line to ride through the Haunted House. John and his brother get into one car. John's mother and father are in another car.

When the ride is over, John and his brother stand outside and wait for their mother and

227

father. They wait and wait. John can't
understand where they could be. John's
brother begins to cry. What should John do?
How can he solve his problem?

The students give answers to the problem, and the teacher
writes the responses on the board.

The activity continues until each student can verbalize an
appropriate solution to a travel-related problem.

<u>MATERIALS</u>:   Chalk; chalkboard; eraser

<u>PROCEDURE 2</u>:

The students are seated in a semicircle facing the chalk-board. The teacher says:

> We have learned many things about traveling.
> Today we are going to solve problems that
> might arise while we are traveling. We will
> "brainstorm." When a group "brainstorms,"
> each group member listens to the problem and
> gives suggestions as to how to solve the
> problem. Here is the first problem.
>
> > John is driving the family car. He
> > is on his way to a job interview.
> > He must arrive on time. He must take
> > a detour. As he follows the detour
> > signs, the car ahead of him stalls.
> > John realizes he will be late to the
> > interview. What should he do?

The teacher and the students "brainstorm" solutions to the problem. The teacher writes all solutions in sentence form on the chalkboard. After he has written the solutions on the board, he says:

> We have many ideas on the board. Let's dis-
> cuss all of the ideas. We can then decide
> which is the best solution to the problem.

After the teacher and students have discussed all solutions and selected the best solution to the problem, the teacher erases the solutions from the board and then presents another travel-related problem to the students.

This activity continues until each student can demonstrate an ability to solve problems that might occur during travel.

<u>Note</u>: The teacher might present problems, such as being lost while traveling, running out of money, having reservations cancelled, getting sick while traveling, misplacing travelers' checks.

OBJECTIVE: Each Student Can Demonstrate an Understanding of the Concept, "Safety," in Regard to Travel

---

MATERIALS: "Safe traveler" badges, one badge for each student; chalk; chalkboard; eraser

PROCEDURE 1:

    (Prior to this activity, the teacher has made "safe traveler" badges from construction paper. There is one badge for each student. Each badge is a different color.)

    The students are seated in a semicircle, facing the chalkboard. The teacher explains:

        Today we are going to talk about safety. You are going to learn ways to make travel safer. I have made a "safe traveler" badge for each of you. To earn your badge, you must be able to name one way to be a safe traveler when you are walking, when you are riding in the car and when you are riding on the bus.

        Let's think of some ways that we might be safe travelers in a car. After you have named a way to make riding in the car safer, I will write it on the board.

        Patty, what is one way to make riding in the car safer?

    Patty responds:

Wear a seat belt.

The teacher says:

> Yes, Patty, we can make riding in the car
> safer by wearing our seat belts. You have
> earned one point toward your safety badge.
> I will write your safety hint on the board.

After each student has named one way to make traveling by
auto safer, the teacher continues:

> Each of you has named one way to make car
> travel safer. Each of you has earned one
> point toward your "safe traveler" badges.
> There are many other ways that we can make
> car travel safer. Can anyone tell us
> another way?

The teacher lists the students' responses on the chalkboard
but does not give additional points for these responses.
The teacher may wish to provide the students with additional
methods of making car travel safer. These methods should be
listed on the board also. The teacher continues:

> We have talked about many ways to make car
> travel safer. Now let's talk about being safe
> travelers when we are walking. I will erase
> the board. While I am erasing the board,
> think of ways we can travel safely while we
> are walking.

After the teacher has erased the material on the board, he
asks the students to contribute their ideas for making
walking safer. The teacher writes the students' ideas on
the chalkboard. It may be necessary for the teacher to assist some students in contributing ideas. Each student is
given one point for contributing to the discussion. The
teacher may provide additional safety tips and lists them
on the board, along with the student responses.

This activity continues until each student has contributed a
safety idea for each of the three types of travel listed and
has received his "safe traveler" badge.

NOTE: To reinforce the idea of how to travel safely, the teacher might invite a guest lecturer, such as a policeman, sheriff or state trooper, to speak to the class. After the talk, the teacher could ask the students to list ways in which they might make travel safer in the three modes of transportation discussed.

MATERIALS: Guest speakers; overhead projector; newspaper articles
             featuring accidents caused by violation of safe driving
             rules

PROCEDURE 2:

(Prior to this activity, the teacher has arranged for a
speaker from the police department, one from the safety
control department of an airline and one from the schools'
department of transportation to speak to the students on
safe traveling. In addition, the teacher has cut articles
from newspapers which report accidents involving cars, buses
or airplanes.)

At the beginning of this activity, each speaker presents his
talk to the class. There is a question-answer and discussion
period following each speech.

At the beginning of the next class period, the students are
seated at their desks, facing the overhead projector. The
teacher remarks:

> We have listened to our guests tell about ways
> to make travel by car, plane and bus safer. I
> have brought articles from the local newspapers
> to class. These are articles about accidents
> which have happened in our city and in other
> cities. I will put the articles on the pro-
> jector and will read them to you. Listen care-
> fully to the stories. You will hear what
> caused the accidents. When I have finished
> reading each of the articles, you may tell
> what caused the accident and how the accident
> could have been avoided. Listen to the first
> article.

The teacher reads the first article to the class. The
teacher continues:

> You have heard the first news story. It was
> a story in which a car crashed into a tele-
> phone pole. Beth, please tell us what hap-
> pened to the driver in the story.

234

Beth responds:

He was thrown from the car.

The teacher asks:

Was he wearing a seat belt?

Beth answers:

No, he wasn't.

The teacher asks:

What caused the accident?

Beth answers:

The driver was speeding. The road was wet.
He lost control of his car.

The teacher comments:

Very good, Beth. You listened carefully to
the story. What safety rules were broken
by the driver?

Beth responds:

He wasn't wearing a seat belt.

The teacher replies:

Yes, Beth, he was not wearing a seat belt.
We should always wear our seat belts in the
car. Seat belts help reduce the severity

of an accident. What other safety rules did the driver break? I can think of two. What are they?

Beth says:

He was speeding. He went too fast on a wet road.

The teacher remarks:

Yes, Beth, he was speeding. He was going too fast for the weather conditions. When the weather is bad or the road is dangerous, we should go slower than the speed limit. Beth, you have told us what caused the accident. You have told us what safety rules were broken. Now, tell us how you might have avoided the accident if you had been the driver.

Beth replies:

I would have worn my seat belt. I would not have speeded. I would have driven slowly on a wet road.

The teacher comments:

Very good, Beth. The accident might have been prevented if the driver had followed those safety rules.

This activity continues until each student has had the opportunity to respond to questions related to the accident articles.

MATERIALS: Stories involving situations in which students may exercise courtesy while they are traveling

PROCEDURE 1:

The students are seated in a semicircle. The teacher begins:

> Today we are going to talk about the word "courtesy." A courteous person is polite. You should be courteous to everyone. You should be courteous at all times. Think of ways you can be courteous at home. Raise your hand when you have thought of ways to be courteous at home.

After several students have named ways to be courteous at home, the teacher asks the students to think of ways that they can be courteous at school. After the students have responded, the teacher remarks:

> You have told ways that you might be courteous at home and at school. You may be courteous travelers also. Each day you travel from one place to another. You often travel by foot, by car, by bus and by bicycle. Today you will think of ways that you might be courteous travelers. When you tell about how you can be courteous travelers, be sure to use sentences.

Listen carefully to our first story. Can you
think of ways that the person in the story
might be a courteous traveler? Here is our
story.

Phil was going to the library. As he
waited for the light to change, he
noticed a lady who was standing behind
him. She was carrying many books. She
had so many books that she dropped one.
She was going to the library too. How
could Phil be a courteous traveler?

Marilyn, how do you think Phil could be a
courteous traveler?

Marilyn replies:

He could help carry the lady's books.

The teacher remarks:

Very good, Marilyn. You have told us one way
that Phil could be a courteous traveler.

Now let's go on to the next story.

After each student can respond appropriately to different
stories involving courtesy while a person is traveling, the
teacher continues:

Now each of you may tell how you might be a
courteous traveler. Remember, use sentences
when you are talking about being a courteous
traveler. Raise your hand when you are ready.

The teacher aids the students in recalling situations in
which they have demonstrated courtesy while they were
traveling. If the students cannot recall such situations,
they can make them up. The teacher reminds them to use
sentences.

This activity continues until each student can demonstrate
an understanding of ways he might show courtesy while he is
traveling.

MATERIALS: Art supplies for making posters (poster board, felt-
tipped markers, magazines, scissors, glue, masking
tape); long table; chalk; chalkboard; eraser

PROCEDURE 2:

(Prior to this activity, the teacher has collected and
assembled art supplies for making posters. These supplies
(poster board, felt-tipped markers, magazines, scissors,
glue, masking tape) have been placed on a long table at the
back of the classroom.)

The students are seated at their desks. The teacher explains:

Today we are going to talk about the word
"courtesy." Who can define "courtesy" for
us? Remember, when we define a word, we tell
what it means.

Raymond, what does "courtesy" mean?

Raymond responds:

"Courtesy" means being polite.

The teacher agrees:

Yes, a courteous person is polite. He is
well-mannered. He is thoughtful of others.
We should try to be courteous at all times.

Now that we know what "courtesy" means, let's
think of ways to be courteous travelers.
Many of you will be driving soon. Some of
you already drive. How can you show courtesy
to others while you are driving? How can you
be thoughtful of others while you are driving?
Raise your hand if you can tell us.

The teacher lists student responses on the chalkboard. When
he has listed all the responses the students can think of,
he continues:

You have mentioned many ways that you might
show courtesy to others while you are traveling. I think you should help make others
aware of ways that they might be courteous
travelers. You may do this by using the
ideas for courtesy to make posters. You
will hang the posters in the halls for all
the students to see.

At the back of the room are some art supplies.
Take the supplies you will need to your desks.
You may use the suggestions on the board for
ideas in creating your posters. If any of
you need help, raise your hand, and I will
come to your desk.

After each student has completed his poster, he may show the
poster to the class and then hang it in the hall for other
students to see.

Note: The teacher may expand this activity by creating
       different units, emphasizing ways that a person might
       demonstrate courtesy while he is walking, riding on a
       bus, driving, flying or using the subway.

OBJECTIVE: **Each Student Can Demonstrate an Understanding of the Concept, "Responsibility," in Regard to Travel**

MATERIALS: Large cardboard numbers, 1 thru 20; large piece of cardboard, divided into four sections across and five sections down; four prizes, which might include pencils, felt-tipped markers, notebooks, erasers or any objects that are readily available and that the students might enjoy

PROCEDURE 1:

(Prior to this activity, the teacher has made large cardboard numbers, 1 thru 20, and has divided a large piece of cardboard into four sections across and five sections down. The teacher has numbered the sections 1 thru 20, first across and then down, and has placed stars behind four of the numbers.)

The students are seated at their desks. The teacher begins the activity by reviewing with the class the concept of responsibility. Then he says:

We have spent several days talking about travel. Today we will talk about being responsible travelers. If each of you can tell us one way to be a responsible traveler while you are walking, you may pick a number from 1 thru 20 on this board. Behind four of the numbers are stars. If you pick a number that has a star behind it, you will win a prize.

John, how can you be responsible while you are traveling on foot?

243

John responds:

> I can cross the street on the green light.

The teacher comments:

> Very good, John. You may pick a number.

After John has picked a number, the teacher remarks:

> John has picked number 2. I will turn over
> number 2. There is no star behind this
> number.
>
> Ann, please tell us another way we can be
> responsible travelers while we are walking.

Ann responds:

> Don't cross in the middle of the street.

The teacher remarks:

> Well done, Ann. You may pick a number.

If Ann picks a number with a star behind it, the teacher
lets her choose a prize.

This activity continues until each student can demonstrate
an understanding of ways to be responsible in regard to
travel.

Note: The teacher may change the mode of travel to include
       riding in a car or school bus, swimming, boating
       and/or flying.

MATERIALS: "Travel agent" badge; box; cards on which the following words are printed, one word per card: "money,"
"car," "bus," "hiking," "skating," "swimming,"
"boating," "skiing," "food," "rest," "exercise";
prize (such as a pencil, a felt-tipped marker, a
notebook, an eraser, etc.); chalk; chalkboard; eraser

PROCEDURE 2:

(Prior to this activity, the teacher has made the "travel
agent" badge and has printed the words on the cards.)

The students are seated at their desks. The teacher introduces the concept of responsibility, in regard to travel.
After the teacher and the students have discussed the concept so that the students understand what it means to be
responsible when they travel, the teacher says:

> John, please take this badge. It says "travel
> agent." You can be the travel agent as long
> as you can tell ways to be a responsible
> traveler. For every way that you mention, I
> will put a checkmark on the board next to
> your name. The person who has the most check-
> marks will win a prize. Are you ready? Pick
> a card from the box.

After John has picked a card from the box, the teacher says:

> You have picked the card that says "money."
> You may tell us all the ways you can be a
> responsible traveler in regard to money.

When John has named all the ways he can be a responsible
traveler in regard to money and has received a checkmark by
his name for each correct response, the teacher remarks:

> Good, John. You have earned seven points. I
> will place the number "7" beside your name on
> the board. Take another card from the box.
> Choose someone to tell how to be a responsi-
> ble traveler.

If John picks the card on which the word "car" is written, the teacher comments:

> You have picked the word "car." You have
> chosen Beth to tell how to be a responsible
> traveler in regard to travel by car. You may
> give her the "travel agent" badge.

The teacher gives Beth a checkmark for each correct response she gives to ways to be a responsible traveler by car.

This activity continues until each student has had an opportunity to demonstrate ways to be a responsible traveler. The student having the most correct responses is awarded a prize.